T0226824

Orofacial Pain

Editor

STEVEN D. BENDER

DENTAL CLINICS OF NORTH AMERICA

www.dental.theclinics.com

October 2018 • Volume 62 • Number 4

ELSEVIER

1600 John F. Kennedy Boulevard ● Suite 1800 ● Philadelphia, Pennsylvania, 19103-2899

http://www.dental.theclinics.com

DENTAL CLINICS OF NORTH AMERICA Volume 62, Number 4
October 2018 ISSN 0011-8532, ISBN: 978-0-323-64121-0

Editor: John Vassallo; j.vassallo@elsevier.com
Developmental Editor: Laura Fisher

Dental Clinics of North America (ISSN 0011-8532) is published quarterly by Elsevier Inc., 360 Park Avenue South, New York, NY 10010-1710. Months of issue are January, April, July, and October. Business and Editorial Offices: 1600 John F. Kennedy Boulevard, Suite 1800, Philadelphia, PA 19103-2899. Periodicals postage paid at New York, NY and additional mailing offices. Subscription prices are $294.00 per year (domestic individuals), $581.00 per year (domestic institutions), $100.00 per year (domestic students/residents), $364.00 per year (Canadian individuals), $751.00 per year (Canadian institutions), $422.00 per year (international individuals), $751.00 per year (international institutions), and $200.00 per year (international and Canadian students/residents). International air speed delivery is included in all *Clinics* subscription prices. All prices are subject to change without notice. **POSTMASTER:** Send address changes to *Dental Clinics of North America*, Elsevier Health Sciences Division, Subscription Customer Service, 3251 Riverport Lane, Maryland Heights, MO 63043. **Customer Service (orders, claims, online, change of address): Elsevier Health Sciences Division, Subscription Customer Service, 3251 Riverport Lane, Maryland Heights, MO 63043. Tel: 1-800-654-2452 (U.S. and Canada). Fax: 314-447-8029. E-mail: journalscustomer service-usa@elsevier.com (for print support); journalsonlinesupport-usa@elsevier.com (for online support).**

Reprints. For copies of 100 or more, of articles in this publication, please contact the Commercial Reprints Department, Elsevier Inc., 360 Park Avenue South, New York, NY 10010-1710. Tel.: 212-633-3874; Fax: 212-633-3820; E-mail: reprints@elsevier.com.

The *Dental Clinics of North America* is covered in *MEDLINE/PubMed (Index Medicus), Current Contents/Clinical Medicine, ISI/BIOMED* and *Clinahl*.

Contributors

EDITOR

STEVEN D. BENDER, DDS
Diplomate, American Board of Orofacial Pain, Clinical Assistant Professor, Department of Oral and Maxillofacial Surgery, Director, Facial Pain and Sleep Medicine, Texas A&M College of Dentistry, Dallas, Texas, USA

AUTHORS

GALIT ALMOZNINO, DMD, MSc, MHA
Department of Oral Medicine, Sedation and Maxillofacial Imaging, Head, Division of Big Data, Department of Community Dentistry, Lecturer, Director, Orofacial Sensory Clinic, Hebrew University-Hadassah School of Dental Medicine, Jerusalem, Israel

PAULA FURLAN BAVIA, DDS, PhD
Division of Oral and Maxillofacial Pain, Department of Oral and Maxillofacial Surgery, Massachusetts General Hospital, Boston, Massachusetts, USA

STEVEN D. BENDER, DDS
Diplomate, American Board of Orofacial Pain, Clinical Assistant Professor, Department of Oral and Maxillofacial Surgery, Director, Facial Pain and Sleep Medicine, Texas A&M College of Dentistry, Dallas, Texas, USA

CHARLES R. CARLSON, PhD, ABPP
Professor, Department of Psychology, Orofacial Pain Clinic, University of Kentucky, Lexington, Kentucky, USA

EDUARDO E. CASTRILLON, DDS, MSc, PhD
Section of Orofacial Pain and Jaw Function, Department of Dentistry and Oral Health, Faculty of Health, Aarhus University, Aarhus, Denmark; Scandinavian Center for Orofacial Neurosciences (SCON)

JANINA CHRISTOFOROU, BDSc(Hons), DClinDent(OralMed/OralPath), FRACDS(GDP), MRACDS(OralMed), FOMAA
Clinical Lecturer, Honorary Research Fellow, University of Western Australia, School of Dentistry, Nedlands, Western Australia, Australia

HAYLEY A. COLE, MS
Clinical Psychology Graduate Student, Department of Psychology, University of Kentucky, Lexington, Kentucky, USA

PAULO CONTI, DDS, MSc, PhD
Professor, Department of Prosthodontics, Bauru School of Dentistry, University of São Paulo, Bauru, São Paulo, Brazil

JEFFREY A. CRANDALL, DDS
Active Staff, Surgery Health Care Service, University of Vermont Medical Center, Burlington, Vermont, USA

SHUCHI DHADWAL, BDS, DMD
Assistant Professor, Department of Diagnostic Sciences, Tufts University School of Dental Medicine, Boston, Massachusetts, USA

FERNANDO G. EXPOSTO, DDS, MSc
Section of Orofacial Pain and Jaw Function, Department of Dentistry and Oral Health, Faculty of Health, Aarhus University, Aarhus, Denmark; Scandinavian Center for Orofacial Neurosciences (SCON)

GIOVANA FERNANDES, DDS, MSc, PhD
Postdoctoral Student, Department of Dental Materials and Prosthodontics, Araraquara School of Dentistry, Univ Estadual Paulitsa, Araraquara, São Paulo, Brazil

GIULIO FORTUNA, DMD, PhD
Assistant Clinical Professor of Oral Medicine, Editor-in-Chief, American Journal of Oral Medicine, Department of Neurosciences, Reproductive and Odontostomatological Sciences, Federico II University of Naples, Naples, Italy

DANIELA A.G. GONÇALVES, DDS, MSc, PhD
Professor, Department of Dental Materials and Prosthodontics, Araraquara School of Dentistry, Univ Estadual Paulitsa, Araraquara, São Paulo, Brazil

ISTVAN A. HARGITAI, DDS, MS
Chairman, Orofacial Pain Center, Naval Postgraduate Dental School, Diplomate, American Board of Oral Medicine, American Board of Orofacial Pain, Bethesda, Maryland, USA

SHEHRYAR NASIR KHAWAJA, BDS, MSc
Orofacial Pain Medicine Consultant, Department of Internal Medicine, Shaukat Khanum Memorial Cancer Hospital, Lahore, Punjab, Pakistan

GARY D. KLASSER, DMD
Professor, Department of Diagnostic Sciences, Louisiana State University Health Sciences Center, School of Dentistry, New Orleans, Louisiana, USA

HUI LIANG, DDS, MS, PhD
Professor, Department of Diagnostic Sciences, Texas A&M University College of Dentistry, Dallas, Texas, USA

ROBERT W. MIER, DDS, MS
Adjunct Instructor, Department of Diagnostic Sciences, Tufts University School of Dental Medicine, Boston, Massachusetts, USA

JEFFRY ROWLAND SHAEFER, DDS, MS, MPH
Division of Oral and Maxillofacial Pain, Department of Oral and Maxillofacial Surgery, Massachusetts General Hospital, Harvard School of Dental Medicine, Boston, Massachusetts, USA

Contents

The assessment, diagnosis, and management of orofacial pain (OFP) disorders is often a complex, multifactorial, and multidisciplinary process. Nociception leads to the perception of pain, causing the personal experience of suffering, which results in pain behavior. Many patients present with various comorbidities that may influence these conditions in a multitude of ways. The clinical presentation of OFP often includes biological, psychological, social, behavioral, and belief system components.

The diagnostic process of pain in the oral, facial, and head region is often perceived as more difficult because of the numerous, extensively innervated structures located in this area. To successfully manage the patient with these pain presentations, it is critical for the clinician to spend ample time procuring a good medical and dental history. A systematic approach to the physical examination will ensure that sufficient data are acquired without overlooking potentially important contributing factors. The use of adjunctive laboratory tests and imaging studies should be based on the findings in the history and examination.

Imaging usefulness in the diagnosis of orofacial pain includes all modalities that cover the soft tissue and bony structures in the region of the head and neck. Imaging techniques may include 2-dimensional and/or 3-dimensional imaging modalities. Both dentists and physicians should be aware of orofacial pain associated with a variety of sources and select the appropriate imaging technique based on the patient's medical and dental history and the clinical examination. The goal of imaging is to provide the clinician with information that will confirm or deny findings of the clinical examination and allow for the selection of an appropriate treatment.

Temporomandibular disorder (TMD), a type of musculoskeletal pain, is the main cause of pain in the orofacial region. It involves the masticatory muscles, temporomandibular joints (TMJs), and associated structures. The most common signs and symptoms are pain, limited range of motion, and TMJ sounds. TMD is a highly prevalent condition with a multifactorial etiology. Management aims to reduce pain and to improve function using a combination of therapeutic options. Noninvasive techniques are the first option and should be indicated considering the needs of each individual, the clinical features, and the mechanisms involved.

Janina Christoforou

Neuropathic pain of the orofacial region can cause much distress in individuals presenting with this condition. It may be easily mistaken for dental pain, and hence many individuals may undergo unnecessary dental work. Knowledge of the types of neuropathic orofacial pain may assist in timely diagnosis and improvement of a patient's quality of life.

Steven D. Bender

Burning mouth syndrome (BMS) is a chronic disorder for which a definitive etiopathology is not known. The patient with BMS often experiences a continuous burning pain in the mouth without any clinical signs. This confusing condition can create frustration for both patient and practitioner. Ultimately, it is important for the practitioner who treats head and face pain to become knowledgeable in the recognition of the many complexities and various presentations associated with BMS. In doing so, the practitioner can be better prepared to help patients cope with this confounding disorder and gain a better quality of life.

Istvan A. Hargitai

Painful oral vesiculoerosive diseases (OVDs) include lichen planus, pemphigus vulgaris, mucous membrane pemphigoid, erythema multiforme, and recurrent aphthous stomatitis. OVD lesions have an immunopathic cause. Treatment is aimed at reducing the immunologic and the following inflammatory response. The mainstay of OVD management is topical or systemic corticosteroids to include topical triamcinolone, fluocinonide, and clobetasol, whereas systemic medications used in practice can include dexamethasone, prednisone, and prednisolone. Oral herpetic lesions can be primary or recurrent. If management is desired, they can be treated by topical or systemic antiviral drugs. Topical antiviral creams include prescription acyclovir, penciclovir, and over-the-counter docosanol.

Robert W. Mier and Shuchi Dhadwal

The primary headaches are composed of multiple entities that cause episodic and chronic head pain in the absence of an underlying pathologic process, disease, or traumatic injury. The most common of these are migraine, tension-type headache, and the trigeminal autonomic cephalalgias. This article reviews the clinical presentation, pathophysiology, and treatment of each to help in differential diagnosis. These headache types share many common signs and symptoms; thus a clear understanding of each helps prevent a delay in diagnosis and inappropriate or ineffective treatment. Many of these patients seek dental care because orofacial pain is a common presenting symptom.

Sleep and pain share a bidirectional relationship. Therefore, it is important for practitioners managing patients experiencing either sleep and/or pain issues to recognize and understand this complex association from a neurobiological perspective involving neuroanatomic and neurochemical processes. Accounting for the influence of pain on the various aspects of sleep and understanding its impact on various orofacial pain disorders assists in developing a prudent management approach. Screening for sleep disorders benefits practitioners in identifying these individuals. Instituting evidence-based multidisciplinary management strategies using both behavioral and pharmacologic strategies enhances the delivery of appropriate care.

Bruxism is an oral behavior that may lead to repetitive jaw-muscle activity characterized by clenching or grinding of the teeth and/or by bracing or thrusting of the mandible with 2 distinct circadian manifestations: sleep bruxism or awake bruxism. They share common risk factors and lead to similar consequences for the masticatory system but may have different etiology and pathophysiology. This oral behavior has been associated with tooth wear, masticatory muscle tenderness, headaches, and painful temporomandibular disorders. Available scientific evidence does not support the view that bruxism is a direct cause of pain, which should be considered when treating/managing patients.

This article examines gender prevalence in orofacial pain to elucidate underlying factors that can explain such differences. This article highlights how gender affects (1) the association of hormonal factors and pain modulation; (2) the genetic aspects influencing pain sensitivity and pain perception; (3) the role of resting blood pressure and pain threshold; and (4) the impact of sociocultural, environmental, and psychological factors on pain.

This article summarizes the cognitive, behavioral, and emotional factors that contribute to the onset and maintenance of orofacial pain. These orofacial pain conditions illustrate the dynamic interplay of the mind and body and the importance of multimodal treatment approaches addressing simultaneously the cognitive, behavioral, and physiologic dimensions of facial pain. Cognitive and behavioral treatments of temporomandibular disorders based on the outcomes of randomized controlled trials are also discussed with an emphasis on using a biopsychosocial perspective when working with the persons who have temporomandibular disorders.

DENTAL CLINICS OF NORTH AMERICA

SERIES OF RELATED INTEREST

Atlas of the Oral and Maxillofacial Surgery Clinics
http://www.oralmaxsurgeryatlas.theclinics.com

Oral and Maxillofacial Surgery Clinics
http://www.oralmaxsurgery.theclinics.com

THE CLINICS ARE AVAILABLE ONLINE!
Access your subscription at:
www.theclinics.com

Preface

Orofacial Pain: Where We Are and Where We Are Going

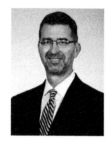

Steven D. Bender, DDS
Editor

It is well known that pain is the primary reason people seek care from their health care providers. The term orofacial pain (OFP) commonly refers to pain associated with the hard and soft tissues of the head, face, oral cavity, and neck. An estimated 25% of the population has experienced some form of OFP, with the highest prevalence in the 18- to 25-year-old age group. OFP may be due to disease of the orofacial structures, musculoskeletal system disorders, peripheral or central nervous system disorders, systemic maladies, the manifestation of psychosocial disorders, or possibly the sequela of poor sleep. OFP can be primary in presentation or secondary due to referral from other sources, such as cervical or intracranial structures. These presentations may include pain of dental origin or of the oral mucosal structures due to infection or inflammation, neurovascular disorders, including poststroke pain, pain from nerve trauma, idiopathic atypical pains, headaches, and finally, disorders of the temporomandibular joints and associated musculature. The diversity of these numerous structures and their complex innervations is at the least partially responsible for the sometimes-puzzling symptoms these patients present with.

In this issue of *Dental Clinics of North America*, it is my hope that the reader not only will be provided with updated information as to the multiple facets of OFP but also will find new information that will further aid them in the diagnosis and management of these often enigmatic disorders. The field of OFP has seen significant progress and change since it was last reviewed in the *Dental Clinics of North America*, both in what we know and in the realization of how needed this specialty is. Also, as our knowledge base has increased, it has become quite clear that the professional who endeavors to diagnose and manage these disorders must commit to look beyond the obvious structures and traditional mechanistic approaches and view the suffering patients as complex and unique individuals who may express pain in very different ways. The clinician must also appreciate the reality that due to the complexity of these

Dent Clin N Am 62 (2018) ix–x
https://doi.org/10.1016/j.cden.2018.08.001
0011-8532/18/© 2018 Published by Elsevier Inc.

patients and the disorders that they present with, a multimodal and multidisciplinary approach to diagnosis and management is critical to positive outcomes. As guest editor, I have purposefully gathered a multinational group of experts in an effort to present a well-balanced and evidence-based treatment of this subject matter. I am extremely grateful to these esteemed contributors for their hard work on this issue. I also wish to express my gratitude to John Vassallo and Laura Fisher for their editorial expertise as well as the entire Elsevier team for their work on this very worthwhile project. I am forever grateful to my father, who always encouraged me to do my very best because "good enough never is." Finally, I wish to thank my best friend and beautiful bride, Micaela, for never giving up on me and hanging in there even though I can't seem to figure out how to spell or pronounce the word "no."

Steven D. Bender, DDS
Department of Oral and Maxillofacial Surgery
Facial Pain and Sleep Medicine
Texas A&M College of Dentistry
3302 Gaston Avenue
Dallas, TX 75246, USA

E-mail address:
bender@tamhsc.edu

An Introduction to Orofacial Pain

Jeffrey A. Crandall, DDS*

KEYWORDS

- Orofacial pain • Comorbidities • Pain processing • Chronic pain
- Temporomandibular disorders • Headache • Neuropathic pain

KEY POINTS

- Orofacial pain (OFP) primarily consists of musculoskeletal, neurovascular, and neuropathic pain conditions.
- Pain processing involves nociception, perception, suffering, and pain behavior.
- These 3 conditions are often accompanied by a variety of comorbidities.
- The clinical presentation of OFP often includes biological, psychological, social, behavioral, and belief system components.

The assessment, diagnosis, and management of orofacial pain (OFP) disorders is often a complex, multifactorial, and multidisciplinary process. The articles in this issue provide the reader with the most current information regarding these conditions and appropriate, evidence-based care for patients who are suffering with these afflictions. In its simplest form, OFP consists of 3 categories: musculoskeletal pain, neurovascular pain, and neuropathic pain. Many of these patients, however, present with various comorbidities that may influence these conditions in a multitude of ways.

In 2014, the National Institutes of Health/National Institute of Dental and Craniofacial Research reported that the prevalence of temporomandibular joint disorder (TMJD) signs and symptoms ranged from 5% to 12%, based on several studies from around the globe.[1] The prevalence of myofascial TMJD in women has been calculated as 10.5% (95% CI, 8.5%–13.0%)[2] and the prevalence of temporomandibular joint (TMJ) osteoarthritis has been found to be 25% in younger adults and as high as 70% in adults over 70 years of age.[3]

A study published in 2010[4] found that 49% of TMJD patients experienced tension-type headaches, 14.5% suffered migraine without aura, 12.9% had probable migraine, 7% suffered migraine with aura, and 4.8% had probable tension-type headaches. Another study of headache patients[5] explored the prevalence of TMJD in

Disclosure Statement: The author has nothing to disclose.
Surgery Health Care Service, University of Vermont Medical Center, 111 Colchester Avenue, Burlington, VT 05401, USA
* 40 Timber Lane, South Burlington, VT 05403.
E-mail address: jacrndl@aol.com

Dent Clin N Am 62 (2018) 511–523
https://doi.org/10.1016/j.cden.2018.05.001
dental.theclinics.com

patients with chronic daily headache and episodic headache. The prevalence of TMJD was found significantly higher in both the chronic daily headache group ($P = .0018$) and the episodic headache group ($P = .05$) when each was compared with the control group. These findings suggest that there is a significant crossover between TMJD and various headaches.

Neuropathic OFP is much more heterogeneous[6] and likely to be a stand-alone diagnosis, as described in an article (See Janina Christoforou's article, "Neuropathic Orofacial Pain," in this issue). As such, the prevalence of each of these disorders is usually independent of the other neuropathic OFP disorders as well as TMJDs and headaches.

PAIN PROCESSING

In many ways, pain affects the entire body but is an experience that occurs within the cortical brain. The process begins with the stimulation of a variety of nociceptors distributed throughout the body and creates neural impulses that are in response to a threat of or real tissue damage.[7] Along with visual, auditory, olfactory, and other stimuli, pain can also create a reflex startle or withdrawal response, in some cases known as hyperexplexia.[8] Ultimately, this may be the generator of a self-protective or so-called fight-or-flight response.

It is beyond the scope of this article to describe the details of the nature of pain. Suffice it to say that nociception leads to the perception of pain, causing the personal experience of suffering, which results in pain behavior. An excellent and detailed description of this process is found in Bell's Oral and Facial Pain.[9] A detailed description and accompanying graphics also is on the Web site, http://neuroscience.uth.tmc.edu/s2/chapter07.html.[10] After the biological phenomenon of nociception, the experiences of perception, suffering, and pain behavior are subject to a broad variety of excitatory and inhibitory influences, also known as the pain modulation concept. Perception of pain is the conscious awareness of an event that has caused tissue damage. But as this awareness becomes more relevant and persistent, the internal emotional response of suffering is initiated. Suffering involves personal and complex interactions between the pain perceiving cortex and the emotional centers, including the thalamus, limbic system, and the reticular activating system. In acute pain, interpreting the magnitude of the tissue damage influences pain behavior. A paper cut generally leads to little or no perceived threat and basic self-care whereas, conversely, more severe trauma results in the immediate search for help. Suffering and pain behavior in the acute model are often accompanied by visible and auditory cues that a person is in distress.

Chronic pain is an altogether different experience and transforms acute pain behavior into a phenomenon that affects mood, work, and social interaction, also known as the biopsychosocial model. Also, conversely, mood, work, and social influences can affect the experience of pain and its interpretation. These patients often present as highly stressed, anxious, and/or depressed and may become hostile. They also may become dependent on family and doctors and can rely on medications and surgeries for treatment. Even the anticipation of pain in the absence of a real stimulus may become a trigger for pain behavior.[11] Fear can become a component of suffering as well, processed through the central nucleus of the amygdala with connections to the thalamus and neocortex.[12] The consequence of chronic suffering may include behaviors, such as avoidance, exaggerated startle response, and hypervigilance, all of which are comparable to posttraumatic stress disorder (PTSD).[13] Thus, when evaluating an OFP patient, it is necessary to consider the influence of the following comorbidities.

COMORBIDITIES: PSYCHOLOGICAL FACTORS

When compared with controls in a study in 2017,[14] TMJD patients experienced greater psychosocial distress. These patients exhibited elevated levels of depression, somatization, and catastrophizing as well as sleep dysfunction. TMJD can lead to chronic pain that is accompanied by a broad variety of psychological disorders, including depression and anxiety. Major depressive disorder is increasingly recognized as a potential component of chronic pain.[15] Acute depression may be the consequence of an abrupt life event, such as a death in the family, and generally improves or resolves within a reasonable period of time. On the other hand, chronic stressful circumstances, such as chronic pain, can lead to long-term and potentially irreversible psychological responses, including major depressive disorder. Prevalence of anxiety disorders, such as PTSD, generalized anxiety disorder, and so forth, has been found 2 times to 3 times greater in chronic pain patients.[16] Acute arousal leads to typical effects on biological responses, such as muscle tension, heart rate, and blood pressure. Chronic arousal, however, can result in long-term alterations in immunologic, neural, and endocrine functions. These factors are significant contributors to a chronic pain patient's pain behavior.

In addition, chronic pain may lead to pain catastrophizing, often found in individuals with sensory over-responsiveness due to a pronociceptive state.[17] The Pain Catastrophizing Scale[18] assesses the role of magnification, rumination, and helplessness as a patient may anticipate or deal with a painful experience. Theoretically, there are at least 4 different mechanisms of catastrophizing. These may include pain appraisal (irrelevant, benign-positive, or stressful-negative), attention bias (pain exaggeration), communal context (secondary gain resulting in reinforcement), and a central mechanism (endogenous pain modulation).[19] These central nervous system and psychological comorbidities result in a vast array of different pain related behaviors that not only have an impact on the individual but also affect family members, friends, work, and social and economic factors in a patient's life. Health care providers need to be cognizant and considerate of all these components of a patient's well-being.

COMORBIDITIES: BEHAVIORAL FACTORS

Oral parafunctional behaviors can include bruxism (clenching and grinding the teeth), biting of oral soft tissues (cheek, lip, and tongue), biting foreign objects (snuff, fingernails, pens, and pencils, and so forth), tooth tapping (eg, to music), and smoking (cigarettes, cigars, and pipes). A search of "oral sexual behavior and TMD" on both PubMed and Google found no relevant results, suggesting that it has not been a topic of research. Although these behaviors may be considered risk factors for the onset of TMJD, they are more likely to be aggravating and perpetuating factors in preexisting forms of TMJD.

Bruxism when awake may often be a response to stressful life events whereas sleep bruxism is recognized by the American Academy of Sleep Medicine as a stereotyped sleep-related movement disorder. The latter should be distinguished from rhythmic mandibular movements associated with sleep disturbances, such as periodic limb movement disorder, arousals, and sleep apnea.[20] A detailed literature review of bruxism found that bruxism when awake occurs predominantly in women whereas bruxism at sleep had no such gender differential.[21]

Relevant to OFP is the additional effect of smoking on pain severity, anxiety, depression, sleep disturbances, and impairment.[22] It has also been found that the prevalence of most TMJD symptoms is greater in those who use snuff and those who consume alcohol more than once per week.[23] Increased caffeine and nicotine intake has been shown to elevate pain-related anxiety in patients with complex regional pain type I without increasing pain intensity.[24]

Drugs of abuse have become a serious concern in the United States and the opioid epidemic has become a significant topic in the media. Patients in pain have a legitimate concern about the management of these symptoms and the impact this has on their well-being. Doctors who treat these patients seek a means of mitigating pain; however, patients may also take matters into their own hands. Patients may obtain pain medications legally through a doctor's prescriptions to a pharmacy but, unfortunately, pain behavior may lead to the acquisition of drugs of abuse from illegal sources. These drugs can lead to an escalation of their TMJD complaints (headache, joint noises, and joint and muscle pain) and increased oromotor behaviors,[25] often unbeknownst to the patients. The medical history for all OFP patients must include information to a patient's exposure to drugs of abuse.

COMORBIDITIES: SLEEP DISORDERS

Obstructive sleep apnea has become a subject of interest and treatment in the dental profession, including the development of organizations focused on the treatment of this condition. The impact of a broad variety of sleep-related disorders, however, on the experience of chronic OFP is much less appreciated. The classification of sleep disorders has been offered by different sources and includes the *International Classification of Sleep Disorders*; the *International Classification of Diseases, Tenth Revision, Clinical Modification*; and the *Diagnostic and Statistical Manual of Mental Disorders* (Fifth Revision).[26] None of these classifications, however, includes specific reference to a pain induced sleep disorder.

It is imperative to understand that sleep has an impact on pain and pain has an impact on sleep, often in a vicious cycle. Svennson and colleagues[27] presented a theoretic and practical perspective about this process, indicating that pain may lead to sleep loss, sleep loss may enhance pain, and sleep loss and pain together can increase pain and sleep loss, and yet the 2 may coexist independent of each other. Choiniere and colleagues[28] have described the relationship between sleep and pain:

- Compared with the general population, sleep disorders are more prevalent in chronic pain patients.
- Patients with chronic pain often report sleep disturbance.
- Insomnia, nonrefreshing sleep, and excessive daytime fatigue are common complaints in chronic pain patients.
- Sleep fragmentation, reduced sleep efficiency, and diminished slow-wave sleep are the most common findings during sleep studies of chronic pain patients.
- Fibromyalgia and other chronic pain conditions produce alpha-delta intrusions during non–rapid eye movement sleep.
- Sleep apnea, restless legs syndrome, and periodic leg movements during sleep are also frequent findings in chronic pain patients.

Because of the close and reciprocal relationship between pain and sleep, the specialty of OFP must be especially cognizant of this influence in a patient's pain complaints.

COMORBIDITIES: HEADACHE DISORDERS

The beta version of the *International Classification of Headache Disorders, 3rd Edition* (*ICHD-3*), includes section 11.7, which describes, "Headache attributed to temporomandibular joint (TMJ) disorder."[29] The description of the diagnostic criteria is based on simplistic premises that the headache:

- Onset occurs at the time as the development of the TMJD
- Increases with the worsening of the TMJD
- Is improved with diminished symptoms of TMJD
- Is worsened by provocation of the TMJD during examination
- Occurs ipsilateral to the TMJD

There is also a comment that headaches due to TMJD may also fit into the classification of *ICHD-3* primary headaches, section 2, "Tension-type headache." The Diagnostic Criteria for Temporomandibular Disorders, published in 2014,[30] also describes "headache attributed to [temporomandibular disorder] TMD" that is consistent with the *ICHD-3* beta version description.

The prevalence of headache in TMJD patients is substantial. A study from Brazil published in 2013[31] found that headache was present in 25.8% of young patients with moderate TMJD and 11.8% of patients with severe TMJD. Chronic daily headache, migraine, and episodic tension-type headache have been found frequent in TMJD patients.[32] Increased headache frequency was associated with increased intensity of TMJD pain. A convergence hypothesis for headache[33] suggests that this pain may progress from a premonitory phase, through tension-type headache, and eventually into migraine. Peripheral nociceptive input from TMD may contribute to the peripheral and central sensitization that leads to this escalation of pain.

COMORBIDITIES: SYSTEMIC DISORDERS

A broad variety of systemic conditions affect the mouth and jaws.[34] Some of these may include pain as a presenting complaint; however, others may result in significant dental and craniofacial skeletal deformities. Progressive malocclusion must be considered a consequence of systemic and behavioral sources when assessing a patient for dental restoration or orthodontics.

Common systemic causes of these conditions include seropositive rheumatoid and juvenile rheumatoid arthritis. There are a broad variety of additional conditions, however, that may affect the TMJ and result in progressive OFP disorders.[35] Spondyloarthritides, connective tissue diseases, and crystal-induced diseases have the potential to create pain, limited jaw range of motion, and TMJ degenerative changes. These OFP conditions may have a substantial impact on a dentist's ability to access the patient's mouth for standard dental care due to pain and limited range of motion. Both the treating dentist and the OFP dentist should cooperatively address a patient's complaints of pain during treatment and postoperatively. In situations such as these, the OFP and craniofacial and dental conditions are the local expression of a systemic condition, and primary management lies within the scope of medical community. The OFP dentist must address a patient's needs in a multidisciplinary manner with the patient's other health care providers.

COMORBIDITIES: TRAUMA

Orofacial trauma is a common contributor to the development of OFP. Those who experience the physical consequences of sports injuries, motor vehicle accidents, accidental falls (eg, from skiing, stairs, and icy conditions) and work-related events (eg, mechanics and caregivers for the emotionally challenged) are subject to the development of acute and subsequently chronic OFP. It is also important to recognize that several events, such as gunshots from failed suicide attempts, trauma from abusive relationships, and unanticipated consequences from dental implant place-ment, can lead to acute and chronic OFP. These events are prone to contribute to a variety of extended emotional sequelae including anger, blame placing, and litigation. Emotional trauma alone (ie, the death of a loved one) may be another potential contrib-utor to the development of OFP. Although the OFP dentist may be focused on a pa-tient's pain complaints, it is also appropriate to encourage counseling for the emotional consequences of these events.

A study in 1995[36] found that 68.9% of OFP patients at an OFP center reported a his-tory of abuse in an anonymous survey whereas only 8.5% reported such abuse in their clinical questionnaire. Another study published in 1996[37] found that patients with a history of childhood sexual abuse were more likely to be hesitant to schedule and attend dental appointments, to experience posttraumatic stress symptoms during dental care, and to experience TMJDs, including bruxism. The insertion of foreign ob-jects into the mouth under these circumstances can also contribute to physical as well as emotional trauma.

In 2007, a study[38] reported that patients with combined TMJD and PTSD symptoms were more likely to experience psychological dysfunction. It was also found that pa-tients with masticatory muscle pain were more likely to experience life interference, af-fective distress, and sleep disturbances than those with TMJ-related pain disorders.

A MODEL OF THE CHRONIC, COMPLEX OROFACIAL PAIN PATIENT

Considering the comorbidities discussed previously, it is appropriate to combine these factors into the development of a diagnostic process that is all-inclusive. **Table 1** is intended to integrate the elements of a patient's biopsychosocial factors combined with behavioral and spiritual (belief system) elements with those events and circumstances that have led to their OFP condition. This includes consideration of the predisposing, precipitating, and perpetuating factors contributing to a patient's complaints, as described by Travell and Simons.[39] In reviewing the diagram from the upper left to the lower right, it is possible to envision how a patient may have pro-gressed over time from an asymptomatic state into chronic, complex OFP. Special emphasis should be placed on the perpetuating risk factors that contribute to the pro-gression into pain chronicity.

Childhood neglect and abuse are common, with a national rate of approximately 9.2 victims per 1000 children in 2012, based on data collected by the Children's Bureau (Administration on Children, Youth and Families; Administration for Children and Fam-ilies) of the US Department of Health and Human Services.[40]

Table 2 presents a theoretic approach to the neuroanatomy and central processing that may contribute to a patient's presentation and complaints. The comorbidities, discussed previously, not only influence but also may alter a broad variety of brain functions, progressing from an acute episode to a long-term but remitting experience to eventually chronic, persistent, and intractable pain. A patient's sense of hopeless-ness and a belief of being incapable of improvement leads to a variety of negative at-titudes and behaviors that may be self-destructive. The consequences can be devastating on a variety of personal, family, and social levels, and self-harm is a distinct possibility. The complexity of neuroscience in the context of the spiritual belief system is presented in a monograph by Felix Larocca.[41]

RISK FACTORS AND PROTECTIVE FACTORS

Considering the broad spectrum of factors that contribute to the onset, development, and progression of chronic, complex OFP, it is necessary to assess the various risk

Table 1
Clinical presentation of the chronic orofacial pain patient

Contributing Factors in Chronic Temporomandibular Disorder and Orofacial Pain	Biological- (Nociception)	Psychological- (Perception)	Social (Suffering)	Behavioral (Physical Response)	Spiritual (Belief Systems)
Predisposing factors	Craniofacial skeletal deformity	History of childhood physical abuse	Childhood in a drug abusive setting	Oral parafunctional habits	Childhood abuse and neglect
Precipitating factors	A blow to the jaw	Terrorized by assault and rape	Intrusive police investigation	Stress from dental treatment, trauma, etc.	External locus: "You did this to me"
Perpetuating factors	Irreversible tissue damage and chronic pain	PTSD, anxiety and depression	Continued drug abuse for chronic pain control	Sleep disorders, bruxism, chronic pain	Hopelessness: unable to improve

Table 2
Theoretic neuroanatomy of the chronic orofacial pain

Contributing Factors in Chronic Temporomandibular Disorder and Orofacial Pain	Biological-(Nociception)	Psychological-(Perception)	Social (Suffering)	Behavioral (Physical Response)	Spiritual (Belief Systems)
Predisposing factors	Catechol-O-methyltransferase: Met/met genotype	Limbic system (emotional reactivity)	Hippocampus and prefrontal cortex (memory)	Inherited activation of the oromotor nucleus	Prefrontal cortex and posterior/superior parietal
Precipitating factors	A-delta pain	Amygdala (fight or flight)	Amygdala (fight or flight)	Activation of the reticular activating system	Prefrontal cortex and posterior/superior parietal
Perpetuating factors	C-fiber pain	Thalamus, midbrain, and pons (anxiety and depression)	Dopamine and the limbic system (addiction)	Chronic cortical arousal	Prefrontal cortex and posterior/superior parietal

factors and protective factors that influence these conditions. These factors each include at least 7 variables: the body, lifestyle, emotions, social elements, spiritual elements, mental status, and the environment. **Fig. 1** represents how these factors interact and can progress from acute pain to a chronic pain state.[42]

The evaluation of OFP patients should include the recognition and understanding of these factors on an individualized basis. Each patient presents various combinations of these risk factors and protective factors and it is essential that this be understood by those who provide care. This analysis leads to a more precise diagnosis and effective treatment plan. In the simpler cases, a careful explanation of the circumstances and self-care may be all that is necessary. In the most complex cases, a careful explanation of the circumstances must be combined with treatment that recognizes all of the variables that have been uncovered in the evaluation and diagnosis. These cases often require a multidisciplinary approach. It cannot be emphasized enough that in all cases a thorough evaluation, complete diagnosis, and careful explanation should be provided for the patient because these are the first steps in successful treatment and/ or management of OFP conditions. Providers of care for OFP patients must understand that TMJ is not a diagnosis.

OROFACIAL PAIN MEDICINE AND ACCESS TO CARE

An article by Julie Beck in *The Atlantic*,[43] published in March 2017, reported on the subject of "Why Dentistry Is Separate From Medicine" during an interview of author, Mary Otto, who has written a book, entitled, *Teeth: The Story of Beauty, Inequality, and the Struggle for Oral Health in America*. The interview raises a question regarding the apparent dichotomy in these professions resulting from the difference in training, clinical practice, organizational differences, third-party insurers, governmental regulations, and access to care. This is particularly relevant in that the stomatognathic system is such a critical component of human anatomy, providing functions, such as deglutition, swallowing, speech, and facial expression. How is it then, that the dental profession has not been considered equivalent to other medical specialties?

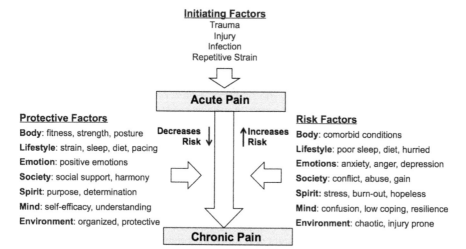

Fig. 1. Interactions of the body, lifestyle, emotions, social elements, spiritual elements, mental status, and the environment.

This article and others like it clearly present the complexity of OFP diagnosis and management. Simply stated, the teeth are the end organ of the gnathic mechanism just as the fingers are the terminus of the arm. Humans use these tools for essential functions of the body necessary for survival. Dentists have been trained to preserve and maintain the teeth but often are poorly educated in the functions of the system that makes them useful. This is comparable to advanced training in treatment of the fingertips while at the same time disregarding the functions of the hand, arm, and shoulder that make them functional. All too often, patients have no means of obtaining evaluation and treatment of their dentition despite access to general health care.

The field of OFP medicine (OFPM) is a link between the medical and dental professions. Many of these patients present with a multitude of medical comorbidities and they frequently require support from a broad variety of medical, psychiatric, and social specialties. Thus, OFP dentists not only provide essential care but also must serve as dental ambassadors to the medical community, sharing knowledge and experience on behalf of these patients as well as learning from medical peers.

OFPM relies on an approach to the whole patient that incorporates problem-oriented medical records.[44] This is a widely used approach that incorporates SOAP notes, referring to a process that includes Subjective information gathering regarding a patient's experience, Objective assessment of a patient's condition (physical examination, laboratory testing, imaging, and so forth), Assessment or diagnosis, and Planning, which leads to a problem list and a course of treatment. This process is essential to establish medical necessity for OFP patients and this is an essential element of access to care. The American College of Medical Quality defines medical necessity as "accepted health care services and supplies provided by health care entities, appropriate to the evaluation and treatment of a disease, condition, illness or injury and consistent with the applicable standard of care."[45]

OFPM must meet the standards of medical necessity if it is to become an accepted part of a patient's overall health care. This also plays a significant role in acceptance by third-party payers, employers who purchase health care insurance, and governmental regulators. It is doubtful that an employer studies and evaluates the quality and limitations of the health care policy being purchased any more than it is likely that the employee/patient studies the policy any time before it is actually needed for a health problem.

IN SUMMARY

As of the time of this writing, the American Dental Association has not included OFPM in its list of recognized specialties. An alternative dental specialty recognition process has been developed, however, by the American Board of Dental Specialties (ABDS). The ABDS recognizes specialty boards that have qualified by submitting a lengthy and detailed application and have satisfied a broad variety of qualifications. The medical profession has long recognized that it is the specialty boards that establish the testing and certification process that lead to the development of a specialty and the ABDS is following this model. The American Board of Orofacial Pain has received full approval from the ABDS, which is currently in the process of obtaining recognition by state boards across the nation. The ABDS represents a viable, alternative pathway for dental specialty certification.

With this activity, it is possible that the field of OFPM will eventually receive the recognition it deserves in the dental and medical communities. Purchasers and providers of health insurance (employers, governmental bodies, and so forth) must recognize the medical necessity of care for these disorders but also must have reassurance that care is efficient and effective. It is the responsibility of the OFPM community of dentists to provide responsible evaluation, diagnosis, and care for patients suffering with these afflictions.

Finally, the Fédération Dentaire Internationale (World Dental Federation) has established a new definition of oral health, stating, "Oral health is multi-faceted and includes the ability to speak, smile, smell, taste, touch, chew, swallow and convey a range of emotions through facial expressions with confidence and without pain, discomfort and disease of the craniofacial complex."[46] As a profession, dentistry is moving beyond the care of the teeth and adjacent tissues, and OFPM has assumed a leadership role in this transition.

REFERENCES

1. Available at: https://www.nidcr.nih.gov/DataStatistics/FindDataByTopic/FacialPain/PrevalenceTMJD.htm. Accessed June 1, 2017.
2. Janal MN, Raphael KG, Nayak S, et al. Prevalence of myofascial temporomandibular disorder in US community women. J Oral Rehabil 2008;35(11):801–9.
3. Das SK. TMJ osteoarthritis and early diagnosis. J Oral Biol Craniofac Res 2013; 3(3):109–10.
4. Kang JK, Ryu JW, Choi JH, et al. Application of ICHD-II criteria for headaches in a TMJ and orofacial pain clinic. Cephalalgia 2010;30(1):37–41.
5. Mello CE, Oliveira JL, Jesus AC, et al. Temporomandibular disorders dysfunction in headache patients. Med Oral Patol Oral Cir Bucal 2012;17(6):e1042–6.
6. Benoliel R, Heir GM, Eliav E. Orofacial pain and headache [chapter 11]. St. Louis (MO): Mosby; 2008. p. 255–94.
7. IASP Task Force on Taxonomy. In: Merskey H, Bogduk N, editors. Classification of chronic pain, second edition. Seattle (WA): IASP Press; 2012.
8. Dreissen YE, Bakker MJ, Koelman JH, et al. Exaggerated startle reactions. Clin Neurophysiol 2012;123(1):34–44.
9. Okeson J. Bell's oral and facial pain. 7th edition. Chicago (IL): Quintessence Publishing; 2014. p. 3–100.
10. Dafny N. Neuroscience online, Department of Neurobiology and Anatomy, University of Texas Health Science Center at Houston, McGovern Medical School. Chapter 7: Pain tracts and sources 1997.
11. Fordyce WE. Behavior conditioning concepts in chronic pain. In: Bonica JJ, editor. Advances in pain research and therapy. vol 5: proceedings of the third world congress on pain. New York: Raven; 1983. p. 781–8.
12. Wirga M. Suffering: its anatomy, physiology and mystique demystified from the nondual medicine perspective. In: Binnebesel J, Formella Z, Krakowiak P, et al, editors. Experiencing a suffering, 1. Rome (Italy): LAS. Libreria Ateneo Salesiano; 2012. p. 3–4.
13. National Institute of Mental Health. Available at: https://www.nimh.nih.gov/health/publications/post-traumatic-stress-disorder-ptsd/index.shtml#pub10. Accessed June 1, 2017.
14. Kothari S, Baad-Hansen L, Svensson P. Psychosocial profiles of temporomandibular disorder pain patients: proposal of a new approach to present complex data. J Oral Facial Pain Headache 2017;31:199–209.
15. Cocksedge Karen SRSC. Depression and pain: the need for a new screening tool. Prog Neurol Psychiatry 2016;20(1):26–31.
16. Asmundson GJ, Katz J. Understanding the co-occurrence of anxiety disorders and chronic pain: state-of-the-art. Depress Anxiety 2009;26(10):888–901.

17. Weissman-Fogel I, Granovsky Y, Bar-Shalita T. Sensory over-responsiveness among healthy subjects is associated with a pro-nociceptive state. Pain Pract 2017. https://doi.org/10.1111/papr.12619. Accessed June 1, 2017.
18. Sullivan MJL, Bishop SR, Pivik J. The pain catastrophizing scale: development and validation. Psychol Assess 1995;7(4):524–32.
19. Quartana PJ, Campbell CM, Edwards RR. Pain catastrophizing: a critical review. Expert Rev Neurother 2009;9(5):745–58.
20. Trindade O, Rodriquez AG. Polysomnographic analysis of bruxism. Gen Dent 2014;62(1):56–60.
21. Shetty S, Pitti V, Satish Babu CL, et al. Bruxism: a literature review. J Indian Prosthodont Soc 2010;10(3):141–8.
22. De Leeuw R, Eisenlohr-Moul T, Bertrand P. The association of smoking status with sleep disturbance, psychological functioning and pain severity in patients with temporomandibular disorders. J Orofac Pain 2013;27:32–41.
23. Mietinen O, Anttonen V, Patinen P, et al. Prevalence of temporomandibular disorder symptoms and their association with alcohol and smoking habits. J Oral Facial Pain Headache 2017;31:30–6.
24. Hsu C, Harden RN, Houle T. Nicotine and caffeine intake in complex regional pain syndrome. J Back Musculoskelet Rehabil 2002;16(1):33–8.
25. Winocur E, Gavish A, Volfin G, et al. Oral motor parafunctions among heavy drug addicts and their effects on signs and symptoms of temporomandibular disorders. J Orofac Pain 2001;15:56–63.
26. Thorpy MJ. Classification of sleep disorders. Neurotherapeutics 2012;9(4):687–701.
27. Svennson P, Baad-Hansen L, Arima T. Association of orofacial pain conditions and sleep disturbance. In: Lavigne G, Cistulli P, Smith M, editors. Sleep medicine for dentists. Chicago (IL): Quintessence Publishing; 2009. p. 167.
28. Choiniere M, Racine M, Raymond-Shaw I. Epidemiology of pain and sleep disturbances and their reciprocal interrelationships. In: Lavigne G, Sessle B, Choiniere M, et al, editors. Sleep and pain. Seattle (WA): IASP Press; 2007. p. 267–84.
29. Olesen J. The international classification of headache disorders, 3rd edition (beta version). Cephalalgia 2013;33(9):627–8.
30. Schiffman E, Ohrbach R, Truelove E, et al. Diagnostic criteria for temporomandibular disorders (DC/TMD) for clinical and research applications: recommendations of the international RDC/TMD consortium network and orofacial pain special interest group. J Oral Facial Pain Headache 2014;28(1):6–27.
31. Branco L, Santis TO, Alfaya TA, et al. Association between headache and temporomandibular joint disorders in children and adolescents. J Oral Sci 2013;55(1):39–43.
32. Goncalves D, Camparis CM, Speciali JG, et al. Temporomandibular disorders are differentially associated with headache diagnoses: a controlled study. Clin J Pain 2011;27(7):611–5.
33. Cady R, Schreiber C, Farmer K, et al. Primary headaches: a convergence hypothesis. headache. The Journal of Head and Face Pain 2002;42:204–16.
34. Kuperstein A, Berardi TR, Mupparapu M. Systemic diseases and conditions affecting jaws. Dent Clin North Am 2016;60(1):235–64.
35. Kononen M, Wenneberg B. Systemic conditions affecting the TMJ. In: Laskin DM, Greene CS, Hylander WL, et al, editors. Temporomandibular disorders, an evidence-based apporach to diagnosis and treatment. Chicago (IL): Quintessence Publishing; 2006. p. 137–46.

36. Curran S, Sherman JJ, Cunningham LL, et al. Physical and sexual abuse among orofacial pain patients: linkages with pain and psychologic disorders. J Orofac Pain 1995;9:340–6.
37. Hays K, Stanley S. The impact of childhood sexual abuse on women's dental experiences. J Child Sex Abuse 1996;5(4):65–74.
38. Bertoli E, de Leeuw R, Schmidt JE, et al. Prevalence and impact of post-traumatic stress disorder symptoms in patients with masticatory muscle or temporomandibular joint pain: differences and similarities. J Orofac Pain 2007;21:107–19.
39. Travell J, Simons D. Myofascial pain and dysfunction, Vol 1: The trigger point manual-upper half of body. Philadelphia (PA): Lippincott Williams & Wilkins; 1998.
40. Available at: http://www.acf.hhs.gov/programs/cb/research-data-technology/statistics-research/child-maltreatment. Accessed June 1, 2017.
41. Larocca, F. The neurosciences of religion: meditation, entheogens, mysticism. Available at: http://www.monografias.com/trabajos59/neurosciences-of-religion/neurosciences-of-religion2.shtml. Accessed June 1, 2017.
42. Fricton J. TMD: comprehensive management [chapter 1]. In: Connelly ST, Tartaglia GM, Silva R, editors. Contemporary management of temporomandibular disorders: current concepts and emerging opportunities. New York: SpringerNature; 2018. p. 1–6.
43. Why Dentistry Is Separate From Medicine. Available at: https://www.theatlantic.com/health/archive/2017/03/why-dentistry-is-separated-from-medicine/518979/?utm_source=atlfb. Accessed August 1, 2017.
44. Mosby. Mosby's medical dictionary. 9th edition. St. Louis (MO): Elsevier; 2009.
45. Poiicy 8. Definition and application of medical necessity: Available at: http://www.acmq.org/policies/policy8.pdf. Accessed August 1, 2017.
46. FDI World Dental Federation. FDS's definition of oral health. Available at: http://www.fdiworldental.org/orla-health/vision-2020/fdisdefinition-of-oral-health.aspx. Accessed August 1, 2017.

Assessment of the Orofacial Pain Patient

Steven D. Bender, DDS

KEYWORDS

- Orofacial pain • Physical examination • Patient assessment • Medical history
- Diagnostic tests

KEY POINTS

- An accurate diagnosis is the key to successful management of the patient with orofacial pain.
- A systematic approach to the gathering of data will help ensure that important aspects of the patient's presenting complaint are not overlooked.
- Adjunctive testing should be driven by the findings in the history and physical examination.
- The psychosocial aspects of the patient's pain presentation cannot be ignored.

INTRODUCTION

As clinicians, one the most important services that we can provide for the patient with orofacial pain is an accurate diagnosis. Many patients with orofacial pain have previously consulted with numerous providers and have received ineffective and, in some cases, inappropriate treatment, based on an incorrect diagnosis. Diagnosis of pain in the oral, facial, and head region is often confounded by the complexity of the numerous, extensively innervated structures located in this area. To effectively manage these patients, a systematic approach to the evaluation process is essential. Along with good history and the patient's description of his or her complaint, a well thought-out comprehensive clinical evaluation is necessary to avoid missing important data relevant to the accurate diagnosis. Additional laboratory tests and imaging studies should be initiated only when deemed necessary to confirm a differential diagnosis formulated from the findings of the history and clinical examination and only if these additional studies will prove to be of significance in developing an evidence-based course of treatment.

THE HISTORY

A comprehensive history will help guide the clinician to conduct the most relevant physical examination. The components of a comprehensive history for the patient

Disclosure Statement: The author has nothing to disclose.
Facial Pain and Sleep Medicine, Department of Oral and Maxillofacial Surgery, Texas A&M College of Dentistry, 3302 Gaston Avenue, Dallas, TX 75246, USA
E-mail address: bender@tamhsc.edu

with orofacial pain include the chief complaint, medical history, dental history, and psychosocial history.

The Chief Complaint

The patient should be given the opportunity to provide the clinician, in his or her own words, a description as to why the patient is seeking care. Other components of the chief complaint should include the following:

Date of onset: "When did your problem start?"
Previous consultations/treatments: "Who else have you consulted with concerning this pain?"
Associated symptoms.
Location: This can be facilitated by diagrams of the head and face for the patient to diagram the areas of pain.
Quality: Validated questionnaires, such as the McGill Pain Questionnaire, can be helpful to evaluate the patient's pain experience.[1] The terms a patient uses to describe the pain can often help the clinician discern the type of pain the patient is experiencing.
Intensity: Verbal or visual scales provide the patient the opportunity to define the intensity of the pain experience using numerical values such as a "0" indicating no pain and a "10" signifying the worst pain imaginable. The intensity of pain also may be expressed as mild, moderate, or severe.
Change over time: Has the pain gotten worse/better?
Aggravating and alleviating factors: What makes the pain worse or helps relieve it?

Past Medical/Dental History

Any illnesses, current or past, should be identified and weighed in relation the patient's present pain experience. Any history of trauma, especially to the head and face, should be documented. Other components of the medical/dental history should include the following:

Medications: past and present (including vitamins and supplements)
Tobacco, alcohol, caffeine, and recreational drug use.
Abuse: physical and/or emotional.
Sleep: quality, snoring, apnea, other disorders.
Dental treatments that may have an impact on the current concern.

A review of systems may reveal systemic entities that are, at least in part, contributing to the patient's pain experience. These may include connective tissue disorders, endocrine disorders, cardiovascular disease, autoimmune disease, and neurologic disorders.

Psychosocial History

Psychosocial factors may play a significant role in the initiation, maintenance, or intensification/chronification of orofacial pain complaints. The psychosocial history will help the clinician understand the patient's mental status and coping skills that may be relevant in eventual therapy recommendations. It is important to include in the history questions concerning depression, anxiety, and stressors, either past or present. The clinician may choose to use validated screeners, such as the 4-item Patient Health Questionnaire (PHQ-4).[2] The important topic of psychosocial aspects in orofacial pain are discussed in detail in Hayley A. Cole and Charles R. Carlson's article, "Mind-Body Considerations in Orofacial Pain," in this issue.

PHYSICAL EXAMINATION

The physical examination should begin with a general inspection of the head and neck, evaluating the general appearance, looking for any evidence of current or previous trauma, asymmetries, swellings, abnormal posture, or involuntary movements. It is preferable to begin the examination positioned in front of the patient. This allows for the opportunity to observe the patient's facial expressions and affect as the process proceeds. It is also facilitates the patient being able to see you. An important part of the evaluation process is to become better acquainted with your patient. Because of the complexity of many orofacial pain complaints, the physical examination also should include an inspection of the ears, both superficially and otoscopically, a nasal examination, and an examination of the oropharynx. Otologic complaints are quite common in the patients who present with temporomandibular disorders.[3] It is useful, especially in patients experiencing a new onset of headache, to include a fundoscopic examination. A neurologic screening, to include a cranial nerve examination, may reveal issues of the nervous system that are either primary or secondary factors to the patient's concern. Other structures to evaluate would include the lymph nodes and vessels to include the carotid, facial, and superficial temporal arteries. Pain to palpation of these vessels may indicate a vascular entity contributing to the pain complaint. Examinations of the masticatory system and the cervical spine as well as an intraoral examination are also necessary components of the comprehensive examination. The masticatory muscles should be palpated and assessed for "familiar pain."[4] This would be pain that is like or similar to the pain that the patient has been experiencing leading to the consultation. Any referral of pain distance from the site of palpation should be noted. It is usually preferable to palpate the selected muscle with one finger, palpating across the muscle fibers (**Fig. 1**).

The suggested force of palpation to apply to masticatory structures is as follows[5]:

1 kg (approximately 2 pounds) at masseter and temporalis muscles (pressure held for 2–5 seconds)
0.5 to 1 kg at the temporomandibular joints
0.5 kg at intraoral sites

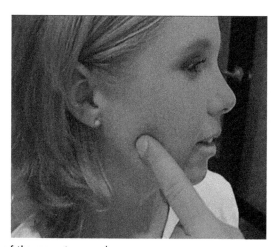

Fig. 1. Palpation of the masseter muscle.

4 kg at neck and shoulder muscles

As the lateral pterygoid muscles cannot be palpated,[6,7] it is necessary to provoke them to assess their status. This can be accomplished by having the patient resist pressure against the action of the muscle (**Fig. 2**).

Along with palpation of the temporomandibular joints to assess for pain, noises emanating from these structures should be recorded as well. It may be helpful to note when the noise occurs during movements, for example, early, middle, or late movement. The noise also can be characterized as to the nature: whether it is a popping noise or more of a crepitus. Joint noises, as well as irregular movements of the mandible, could indicate internal derangements or pathology of the structures. However, it is important to note that these noises do not necessarily correlate with the pain presentation, nor do they provide an indication for therapeutic intervention.[8]

A normal range of motion of mandibular depression is approximately 40 to 50 mm[9] (**Fig. 3**). Lateral and protrusive excursive movements of more than 7 mm are considered to be normal[9] (**Figs. 4** and **5**). It is helpful to ascertain the maximum movement without pain as well as the full maximum movement the patient is capable of. This is termed the active range of motion. In some cases, measuring the maximum movement assisted by the clinician can provide additional helpful data. This measurement is termed the passive range of motion. Noting the location and intensity of the patient's pain during these movements should be a part of the physical examination.

The intraoral examination should be guided by the presenting complaint and history. The soft tissues should be inspected for lesions, suspicious swellings, masses, or ulcerations. Scalloping of the lateral tongue borders may be suggestive of bruxism or sleep-disordered breathing.[10,11] The presence of tori may also suggest bruxism.[12] Wear faceting of the dentition is a common finding suggestive of parafunctional habits that may contribute to the patient's complaint. Although the role of occlusal factors in orofacial pain disorders lacks scientific creditability,[13] relationships should be documented as a part of the comprehensive examination to monitor for any changes due to disease progression during the therapeutic process or with observation. Any so-called "ideal occlusion" is an entity rarely found in nature.[14] If the patient's pain complaint mimics pain of odontogenic origin, appropriate studies, such as pulp vitality testing, radiographic surveys, percussion, and thermal response testing should be used. Milking of the parotid, submandibular, and sublingual glands can assess gross

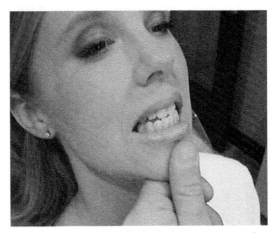

Fig. 2. Provocation to assess the status of the lateral pterygoid muscles.

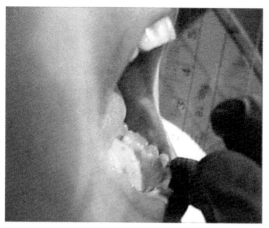

Fig. 3. Measurement of maximum opening.

salivary function. Dabbing the area of the minor salivary glands on the lips and palate with a cotton square and observing the response can determine their status.

DIAGNOSTIC TESTS

The purpose of a diagnostic test is to establish the presence (or absence) of disease as a basis for treatment decisions in symptomatic individuals. All diagnostic tests are not indicated for every patient presenting with orofacial pain complaints. The application of the diagnostic test must be based on the individual's unique presentation after a comprehensive history and physical examination have been performed and the results contemplated. Also, the value of the test should be weighed against evidence-based protocols. Before testing, one must consider if the test will have a meaningful impact on the diagnosis and subsequent course of treatment. If the test does not fulfill these criteria, it should not be ordered. Testing methods for orofacial pain complaints include imaging, laboratory studies, adjunctive electrodiagnostic tests, and diagnostic analgesia. Imaging in orofacial pain is covered in detail in Hui Liang's article, "Imaging in Orofacial Pain," in this issue.

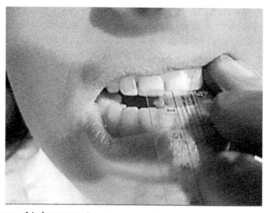

Fig. 4. Measurement of left protrusive movement.

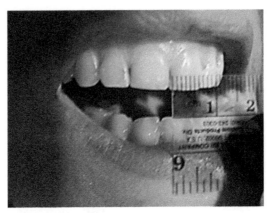

Fig. 5. Measurement of lateral movement.

Only a brief discussion of laboratory test, adjunctive electrodiagnostic studies, and diagnostic analgesia is included, as it is beyond the scope of this article to discuss these topics in detail.

Laboratory Tests

Laboratory tests should not be considered as a routine part of the patient with orofacial pain evaluation. The test should be ordered only to evaluate for certain conditions. These tests may be used to rule in/out metabolic disorders, autoimmune disorders, hematologic disorders, and endocrine disorders. If a sleep disorder is suspected, appropriate screening and testing is recommended. The orofacial pain clinician always should be amenable to consulting with appropriate specialists should suspected disorders fall outside the clinician's expertise or scope of practice.

Adjunctive Electrodiagnostic Tests

First and foremost, any diagnostic test used for the patient with orofacial pain should prove to be both valid and reliable. In addition, the sensitivity and specificity parameters should be known. Sensitivity refers to the ability of the test to accurately identify a condition in a person who has been confirmed to have the condition. The specificity of a particular test refers to its ability to accurately rule out a condition in an individual who does not have the disorder. If a healthy person is identified with a test to have a particular disorder when the person in fact does not, this is referred to as a false positive. With orofacial pain conditions, it is important that diagnostic tests have a great degree of specificity to avoid overdiagnosis and treatment. To date, the use of electrodiagnostic equipment for the diagnosis of orofacial pain lacks sufficient evidence to support its routine use in clinical practice.[15–18]

Diagnostic Analgesia

In select cases of diagnostic uncertainty, the use of local anesthetics can provide invaluable information as to the source of the presenting complaint. The basic premise is if one injects local anesthesia into an area that the patient is reporting as painful and the pain is not relieved, the possibility exists that this area is not the source of the presenting complaint. This technique can be an important tool in discerning referred pain conditions, as well as educating the patient as to this phenomenon. Diagnostic anesthesia also can be used if one is not certain as to whether or not a pain complaint is of masticatory muscle or temporomandibular joint origin. To safely use diagnostic analgesia into clinical practice, it is imperative that the clinician is well versed in anatomy of the head, face, and oral cavity, as well as the nature of the local anesthetic being used. For extraoral anesthetic blocks, strict aseptic techniques must be used. Finally, the decision to use diagnostic anesthesia should be driven by the information gained in the history and physical examination, and the results interpreted based on the same.

SUMMARY

One of the most challenging yet rewarding services we can provide in clinical practice is to successfully diagnose and manage a patient experiencing some form of orofacial pain. Pain in the oral, facial, and head region can provide very unique challenges due to the convergence of afferent information received from these structures into the central nervous system. The evaluation process should begin with allowing the patient to tell his or her story in his or her own words. Additional information can be gained from a comprehensive medical and dental history, including the results of any previous consultations and therapies for the patient's chief concern. It is of equal importance to assess for any psychosocial factors that may be relative to the patient's pain presentation. The examination process should be crafted in such a way as to ensure that all potentially contributing factors are not forgotten. Ideally, we should determine the necessity for any adjunctive diagnostic test, such as imaging and laboratory studies, from the findings of the history and physical examination. Ultimately, it is key to remember that no 2 patients are alike. Each individual will present with very unique aspects to their disorders. The clinical assessment process should not only serve as a data-gathering process, but also as a means to become better acquainted with the individual we hope to help.

REFERENCES

1. Melzack R. The McGill pain questionnaire: major properties and scoring methods. Pain 1975;1(3):277–99.
2. Kroenke K, Spitzer RL, Williams JB, et al. An ultra-brief screening scale for anxiety and depression: the PHQ-4. Psychosomatics 2009;50(6):613–21.
3. Chole RA, Parker WS. Tinnitus and vertigo in patients with temporomandibular disorder. Arch Otolaryngol Head Neck Surg 1992;118(8):817–21.
4. Schwarzer AC, Derby R, Aprill CN, et al. The value of the provocation response in lumbar zygapophyseal joint injections. Clin J Pain 1994;10(4):309–13.
5. Schiffman E, Ohrbach R, Truelove E, et al. Diagnostic criteria for temporomandibular disorders (DC/TMD) for clinical and research applications: recommendations of the international RDC/TMD consortium network* and orofacial pain special interest group†. J Oral Facial Pain Headache 2014;28(1):6–27.
6. Stratmann U, Mokrys K, Meyer U, et al. Clinical anatomy and palpability of the inferior lateral pterygoid muscle. J Prosthet Dent 2000;83(5):548–54.
7. Johnstone DR, Templeton M. The feasibility of palpating the lateral pterygoid muscle. J Prosthet Dent 1980;44(3):318–23.
8. Tallents RH, Hatala M, Katzberg RW, et al. Temporomandibular joint sounds in asymptomatic volunteers. J Prosthet Dent 1993;69(3):298–304.
9. de Wijer A, Lobbezoo-Scholte AM, Steenks MH, et al. Reliability of clinical findings in temporomandibular disorders. J Orofac Pain 1995;9(2):181–91.
10. Sapiro SM. Tongue indentations as an indicator of clenching. Clin Prev Dent 1992; 14(2):21–4.

11. Tomooka K, Tanigawa T, Sakurai S, et al. Scalloped tongue is associated with nocturnal intermittent hypoxia among community-dwelling Japanese: the Toon Health study. J Oral Rehabil 2017;44(8):602–9.

12. Navaneetham A. Lingual bony protruberances—a retrospective analysis. J Indiana Dent Assoc 2010;4(12):603–4.

13. Manfredini D, Lombardo L, Siciliani G. Temporomandibular disorders and dental occlusion. A systematic review of association studies: end of an era? J Oral Rehabil 2017;44(11):908–23.

14. Woda A, Vigneron P, Kay D. Nonfunctional and functional occlusal contacts: a review of the literature. J Prosthet Dent 1979;42(3):335–41.

15. Manfredini D, Cocilovo F, Favero L, et al. Surface electromyography of jaw muscles and kinesiographic recordings: diagnostic accuracy for myofascial pain. J Oral Rehabil 2011;38(11):791–9.

16. Manfredini D, Bucci MB, Montagna F, et al. Temporomandibular disorders assessment: medicolegal considerations in the evidence-based era. J Oral Rehabil 2011;38(2):101–19.

17. Sharma S, Crow HC, McCall WD Jr, et al. Systematic review of reliability and diagnostic validity of joint vibration analysis for diagnosis of temporomandibular disorders. J Orofac Pain 2013;27(1):51–60.

18. Manfredini D, Cocilovo F, Stellini E, et al. Surface electromyography findings in unilateral myofascial pain patients: comparison of painful vs. non painful sides. Pain Med 2013;14(12):1848–53.

Imaging in Orofacial Pain

Hui Liang, DDS, MS, PhD

KEYWORDS

- Imaging • Orofacial pain • Intraoral • Temporomandibular disorder • Neuropathic
- Headache

KEY POINTS

- Imaging in orofacial pain involves using either a 2-dimensional and/or 3-dimensional modality. Each modality has its advantages and disadvantages.
- The diagnosis of orofacial pain challenges both dentists and physicians. For dentists, evaluation of orofacial pain must go beyond the oral cavity, teeth and their supporting structures, temporomandibular joints, and muscles of mastication. Physicians need to rule out common dental-related diseases.
- Imaging usefulness in the diagnosis of intraoral pain disorders, temporomandibular disorders, neuropathic pain disorders, and headaches is discussed.
- Inadequate radiographic evaluation before a dental surgical procedure is the most common cause of trigeminal nerve damage.
- Both dentists and physicians should be aware of pain associated with Eagle syndrome. It is important to remember that the location or site of orofacial pain is not always related to the source of the pain.

INTRODUCTION

The term orofacial pain refers to pain related to soft or hard tissues of the head and neck. It may present as either an acute or a chronic condition. Acute pain begins suddenly and usually does not last long, whereas chronic pain may last longer than weeks or months.[1] Chronic orofacial pain can have a negative effect on the patient's daily activities and quality of life, including sleep, absence from work, or loss of employment.[2] Studies have reported that the prevalence of orofacial pain may vary from 5% to 57% depending on many factors. These factors include the sociocultural differences of the study population, dental awareness of the patient, and the patient's access to dental care.[3,4] The source and pathophysiology of orofacial pain include dental, mucosal, musculoskeletal, neurovascular, and neuropathic.[5] These structures in the head and neck region, along with their complex cranial nerve innervation, make a differential diagnosis of orofacial pain more challenging because of the wide range of diagnostic

Disclosure Statement: The author has nothing to disclose.
Department of Diagnostic Sciences, Texas A&M University College of Dentistry, 3302 Gaston Avenue, Dallas, TX 75246-0677, USA
E-mail address: hliang@tamhsc.edu

Dent Clin N Am 62 (2018) 533–551
https://doi.org/10.1016/j.cden.2018.05.003
dental.theclinics.com

possibilities.[1] Oberoi and colleagues[4] have found that several studies have a similar distribution of orofacial pain symptoms. They showed that toothache was the most common symptom followed by temporomandibular joint (TMJ) pain. Another study used a systematic random sampling of 1668 patients visiting 100 general dentists and concluded that dentoalveolar and musculoligamentous pain were the most prevalent types of pain.[3]

The diagnosis of orofacial pain challenges both dentists and physicians. For dentists, evaluation of orofacial pain must go beyond the oral cavity, teeth and their supporting structures, TMJs, and muscles of mastication.[6] Physicians need to rule out common dental-related diseases. A cross-sectional study conducted in 2016 included 166 general dentists.[7] This study found that dentists had a less than desirable knowledge of the cause of chronic orofacial pain (48.2%), and its clinical presentation (45.2%). Furthermore, only 36.1% had good knowledge of what a physical examination for orofacial pain could include and only 7.8% had good knowledge of how it can be treated. The investigators recommended that educational programs in academic curricula be included to improve general dentists' knowledge of chronic orofacial pain. The diagnosis of orofacial pain bridges an important gap between dentistry and medicine. A multidisciplinary team approach has been recommended to recognize the clinical presentation of orofacial pain, improve treatment outcomes, and prevent the negative impact on the patient's quality of life.[2]

Imaging in orofacial pain involves using either a 2-dimensional and/or a 3-dimensional modality. The selection criteria of imaging modality should be based on the patient's chief complaint and individual needs, and the results of the clinical examination. The use of imaging is to determine the presence and/or absence of disease, to assess the extent and nature of disease, to evaluate the location, and to establish a baseline on which to measure the results of treatment or other intervention. The ultimate goal is to maximize diagnostic efficiency while minimizing patient's radiation risk.

MOST COMMON IMAGING MODALITIES FOR OROFACIAL PAIN

1. Two-dimensional
   a. Intraoral radiography
      i. Periapical radiography
      ii. Bitewing examination
      iii. Occlusal radiography
   b. Extraoral radiography
      i. Panoramic radiography
2. Three-dimensional
   a. Cone beam computed tomography (CBCT)
   b. Multidetector computed tomography (MDCT)
   c. Magnetic resonance imaging (MRI)

The advantages and disadvantages of most common imaging modalities are listed in **Table 1**.

Intraoral Radiography

Intraoral radiography is the most frequently used modality for demonstrating the condition of teeth and their supporting structures. There are 3 categories of intraoral radiographs: periapical, bitewing, and occlusal projections.

- After the clinical examination, periapical radiographs should be made to demonstrate the entire tooth and the surrounding bone in the area of interest. Periapical

Table 1
The advantages and disadvantages of most common imaging modalities

Advantages	Disadvantages
Intraoral periapical and bitewing radiography	
Widely available	Two-dimensional image without facial/
High image resolution	lingual dimension
Minimal magnification	Limited dentoalveolar region
Inexpensive	Limited reproducibility
Low radiation risk	Highly operator dependent
Panoramic radiography	
Commonly available	Two-dimensional image without facial/
Broad anatomic coverage	lingual dimension
Relatively low cost	Moderate image resolution
Low radiation risk	Sensitive to patient positioning errors
Special conditions for trismus or gagging	Inconsistent magnification
patients	Limited for severe maxillofacial discrepancy
CBCT	
Easy to use	Image noise
Less cost compared with CT	Poor soft tissue contrast
Smaller physical size	Artifacts created by metal objects
Fast acquisition	High cost compared with two-dimensional
Submillimeter resolution	images
Relatively low radiation risk compared with	
CT	
Interactive analysis	
MDCT	
Evaluation of large area	Limited availability
Minimum of superimposition	Sensitive to technique errors
Uniform magnification (1:1)	Artifacts created by metal objects
Provides for accurate measurements	Special training needed for interpretation
Bone density evaluation	High cost
Simulates implant placement with software	High radiation risk
MRI	
Painless	High cost
Noninvasive	Limited availability
Soft tissue differentiation	Long acquisition time
No ionizing radiation	Contraindicated for claustrophobic patient
	and patient with pacemaker

radiographs are commonly used for odontogenic pain associated with dental disease either attributed to pulpal (**Fig. 1**) or periodontal origin (**Fig. 2**). Most common dental diseases are dental caries and periodontal disease, the cause of which can be bacterial, traumatic, or iatrogenic. Negative findings on a periapical radiographic examination may rule out orofacial pain of pulpal or periodontal origin. Nonodontogenic pain can be referred or radiated to teeth and their supporting structures.

- Bitewing radiographs demonstrate the crowns of teeth and adjacent alveolar crests. They are considered the best radiographic examination for the diagnosis of interproximal caries (**Fig. 3**) and for the evaluation of the height of interproximal alveolar bone.
- Occlusal radiographs should be made if a relatively large area of the dental arch needs to be visualized in the buccal/lingual dimension and a 3-dimensional study

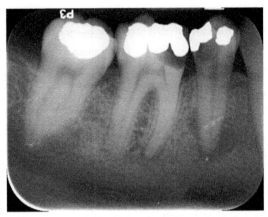

Fig. 1. A right mandibular periapical radiograph shows recurrent caries on the distal and apical periodontitis associated with the premolar tooth and recurrent caries on the mesial of the first molar with apical periodontitis at the apex of the mesial root.

is not available. In addition, occlusal radiographs are made when patients are unable to open wide enough for periapical radiographs in cases of trauma, or to confirm or rule out the presence or absence of a salivary gland stone (**Fig. 4**). Digital intraoral systems most commonly have a sensor size 1 and 2, but size 4 is rarely available. As a result, occlusal radiography has been replaced by a 3-dimensional imaging modality such as CBCT.

Panoramic Radiography

Panoramic radiography is an extraoral technique that can be used as an excellent screening tool because of its broad anatomic coverage of maxillofacial bone and teeth. It is the most commonly used extraoral modality in dental practice. It can be used to investigate orofacial pain that is related to the following:

- Dental pain associated with infections such as pulp disease, periapical abscess, periodontal disease, and osteomyelitis (**Fig. 5**)

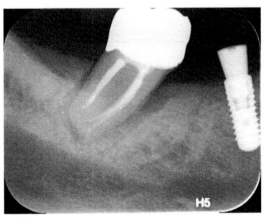

Fig. 2. A 61-year-old man presented with periodontal pain, and a clinically draining sinus tract associated with right mandibular molar. An intraoral radiograph showed horizontal and vertical bone loss. The tooth was previously treated endodontically.

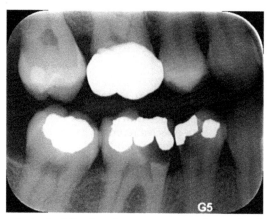

Fig. 3. A right premolar/molar bitewing shows recurrent caries on the distal of the mandibular premolar and mesial surface of the first molar.

- Any intraosseous pathologic condtion that presents with destruction of maxillofacial bone resulting from odontogenic or nonodontogenic cysts or tumors (**Fig. 6**)
- Dentomaxillofacial trauma, such as fracture of the crown and root of teeth, alveolar bone, or the maxillary and mandibular jaws
- Postsurgical infection or trauma following tooth extraction or implant placement procedures
- Either panoramic radiography or CBCT may be necessary in the diagnosis of pain associated with an elongated styloid process or ossification of the stylohyoid ligament
- Research diagnostic criteria for temporomandibular disease do not list panoramic radiography as an imaging modality for evaluation of the TMJ. Panoramic radiography only depicts the lateral poles and central part of the condyle and cannot provide subtle osseous or soft tissue changes. Only advanced bony changes such as rheumatoid arthritis, loose radiopaque TMJ bodies (**Fig. 7**),

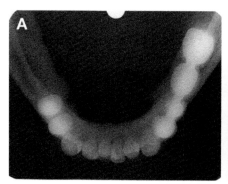
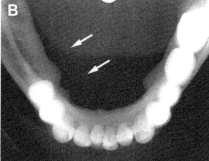

Fig. 4. Radiographs of a 63-year-old man with a 2-day history of pain and swelling in the right floor of mouth. (*A*) A digital mandibular occlusal radiograph without postprocessing and (*B*) with postprocessing shows sialoliths (*arrows*) in the right submandibular gland duct (Wharton duct).

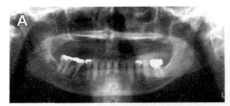
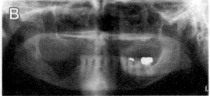

Fig. 5. (A) A 49-year-old woman presented with numbness and pain on her lower right lip and chin. A panoramic radiograph revealed recurrent dental caries on the distal of right mandibular first molar and osteolytic and uneven sclerotic changes in the right mandibular posterior, angle, and ramus. A biopsy returned the finding of osteomyelitis. (B) Eight months after extraction, debridement, and antibiotic treatment, a panoramic radiograph demonstrated normal cortical and trabecular bone with a bony defect in the right mandibular molar region.

traumatic disturbances of joints, or development disturbances of the TMJ can be identified in panoramic radiography[8]

Cone Beam Computed Tomography (CBCT)

Since the introduction of CBCT to dentistry in 1998,[9] this 3-dimensional imaging modality has played a significant role in dental diagnostic sciences. With its increasing availability in private dental practice and imaging centers, there are now numerous CBCT applications that are helpful in a multitude of dental disciplines. Although the "field of view" and "resolution" vary by different CBCT scanners, CBCT can be used to investigate orofacial pain that is related to the following:

- Preimplant and postimplant site evaluation, such as implant-related nerve injury (**Fig. 8**)
- Root morphology and anatomic structure near the apices of teeth (**Fig. 9**)
- Internal/external resorption and the location and position of impacted teeth (**Fig. 10**)
- Dentomaxillofacial trauma, such as fracture of the crown and root of teeth, alveolar bone, or the maxillary and mandibular jaws (**Fig. 11**)
- The morphology of the TMJ
- Mandibular third molar position relative to the inferior alveolar canal
- Maxillofacial pathoses involving the nasal cavity, paranasal sinuses (**Fig. 12**), salivary gland (**Fig. 13**), maxilla, and mandible

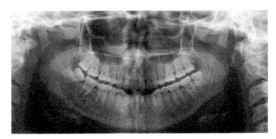

Fig. 6. A 17-year-old woman presented with a large radiolucent and multilocular lesion in the right mandibular molar region. The straight, thin septa within the lesion give it a tennis racket–like appearance. These radiographic findings and location are characteristic of odontogenic myxoma. A biopsy confirmed this diagnosis.

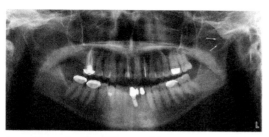

Fig. 7. A panoramic radiograph of a 50-year-old woman revealed multiple radiopaque bodies in the area of the left condyle (*arrows*).

Multiple updated position papers provide guidelines for the use of CBCT in dentistry.[10–13] CBCT can be used for the diagnosis of orofacial pain of either odontogenic or nonodontogenic origin. A review of 26 publications on CBCT between 2000 and 2014 by Horner and colleagues[14] in 2015 reported that 11 were specifically written to present guidelines on the clinical use of CBCT. Of these 11 publications, 2 had used a formal evidence-based approach, 2 used consensus methods, and 7 reported on expert opinions. Generally, there was broad agreement between these guidelines on the clinical use of CBCT in multiple disciplines in dentistry, but variations present in treatment planning for implant dentistry.[14]

Multidetector Computed Tomography (MDCT)

The first CT scanner that used a single detector was developed in England in 1971 for imaging the brain. Since then, in the evolution of today's computed tomographic (CT) scanner, there have been many changes. Scanners have been developed with an

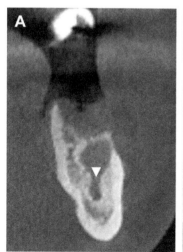
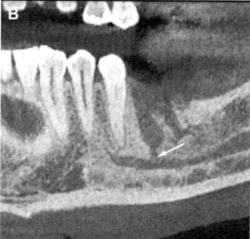

Fig. 8. A 30-year-old woman developed paresthesia 2 weeks following extraction of the left mandibular first molar and placement of a bone graft. After removal of the bone graft, a CBCT study revealed (*A*) a communication between the extraction socket and inferior alveolar canal (*arrowhead*) in the cross-sectional image. (*B*) A cropped pseudopanoramic image showed what appeared to be a bone graft fragment that appeared to have compressed the inferior alveolar canal (*arrow*).

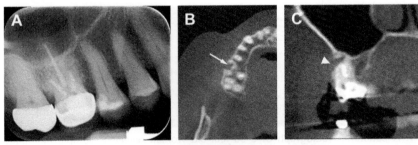

Fig. 9. (A) Intraoral periapical radiograph of a 68-year-old woman showed an endodontically treated maxillary right molar with no periapical radiolucent lesion visible. However, a CBCT study of cropped axial image (B) demonstrated mesial buccal root resorption (*arrow*) and cropped coronal image (C) demonstrated perforation of the buccal cortex (*arrowhead*).

increase in the number of detectors to more than 2000 and a decrease in the scan time from minutes to a few seconds. This modality is frequently and widely used in medical and dental fields because CT images allow radiologists to identify internal structures in 3 dimensions and see their shape, size, density, and texture. CT has less of a signal-to-noise ratio compared with CBCT and as a result a higher quality of image. It offers both a "bone window" and "soft tissue window" to enhance one at the expense of the other. In addition, intravenous contrast agents can be used to enhance soft tissue and vascular image details. CT angiography can provide information regarding carotid flow if stroke or arterial dissection is suspected. CT may be helpful in determining the origin of orofacial pain that is related to the following:

- Head, face, and neck trauma
- The TMJ (**Fig. 14**)
- Infections, cysts, and benign and malignant tumors of head and neck
- Maxillofacial pathoses, involving the nasal cavity, paranasal sinuses, salivary gland, maxilla, and mandible
- Headaches

Magnetic Resonance Imaging (MRI)

MRI was introduced in the early 1980s. This imaging modality that is free from ionizing radiation is capable of showing soft tissue such as nerve and muscle. MRI can provide excellent soft tissue differentiation. It is one of the most authoritative of examinations

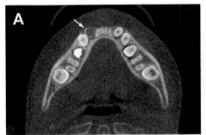
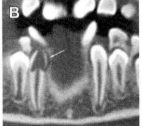
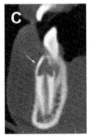

Fig. 10. A CBCT study of a 10-year-old girl shows preeruption intracoronal resorption of the right mandibular canine (*arrow*). (A) CBCT axial image. (B) Cropped pseudopanoramic slice. (C) Cross-sectional image of right mandibular canine.

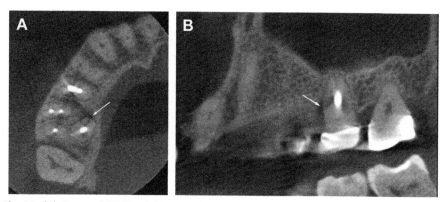

Fig. 11. (A) Cropped CBCT axial image shows a mid root fracture of the mesial surface of the palatal root of the maxillary right first molar (*arrow*). (B) Cropped sagittal image shows localized severe bone loss at mesial surface of the palatal root of the first molar (*arrow*).

and the gold standard for soft tissue pathologic condition, such as a brain tumor. Although MRI, CBCT, or CT can evaluate osseous changes, CBCT or CT is a better choice if bony alterations need to be evaluated. Traditional imaging protocols include T1-weighted and T2-weighted images. MRI can be used to investigate orofacial pain that is related to the following:

- Musculoskeletal disorders
- TMJ disc position and joint shape, the presence of arthritis, and tumors (**Fig. 15**)
- Neurovascular lesions
- Lesions of neuropathic origin

IMAGING MODALITY SELECTIONS FOR OROFACIAL PAIN

The fifth edition[6] of the American Academy of Orofacial Pain guidelines in assessment, diagnosis, and management of orofacial pain has detailed discussion of 7 physical orofacial pain conditions, as follows:

- Vascular and nonvascular intracranial disorders
- Primary headache disorders
- Neuropathic pain disorders
- Intraoral pain disorders
- Temporomandibular disorders

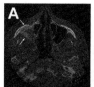
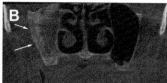
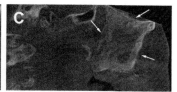

Fig. 12. A CBCT study of a 64-year-old patient with chronic rhinosinusitis shows opacification of the right maxillary sinus with thickened bony walls (*arrows*), without expansion of sinus. (A) CBCT axial image. (B) Cropped coronal image. (C) Cropped sagittal image of the right maxillary sinus.

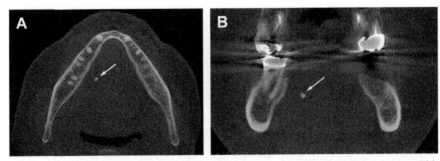

Fig. 13. A CBCT study of a 65-year-old man who presented with pain in the right mandible. (*A*) Axial and (*B*) coronal views show a submandibular gland sialolith (*arrow*).

- Cervical pain disorders
- Extracranial and systemic causes of orofacial pain

However, only 4 of these categories are discussed here for imaging modality selections because of their common occurrence in dentistry and medicine, and their close relationship and presentation in a 2-dimensional and/or 3-dimensional imaging modality. The 4 categories are as follows:

- Intraoral pain disorders
- Temporomandibular disorders
- Neuropathic pain disorders
- Headaches

Intraoral Pain Disorders

The most common orofacial pain is intraoral, involving the teeth and their supporting structures.[4] Orofacial pain may be odontogenic or nonodontogenic in origin, or the result of painful soft tissue oral lesions. More than 95% orofacial pain results from odontogenic origin.[15] The imaging modalities commonly used include intraoral radiography, panoramic radiography, and CBCT. Some complex cases may be further investigated using CT or MRI. **Table 2** lists the most common intraoral pain disorders with selected imaging modalities and radiographic appearance.

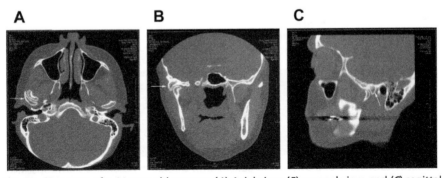

Fig. 14. CT images of a 44-year-old woman. (*A*) Axial view, (*B*) coronal view, and (*C*) sagittal view. The images show an osseous mass (*arrow*) located lateral-posteriorly to the right condyle. A biopsy confirmed an atypical location for a benign osteoma.

A **B**

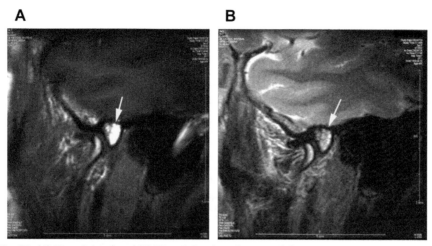

Fig. 15. (A) T1-weighted and (B) T2-weighted MR images of the same patient as **Fig. 14**. The osseous mass demonstrated a marrow signal intensity (*arrow* in A) on the T1-weighted sequences with a low signal peripheral rim (*arrow* in B). This is consistent with cortical bone as shown in the T2-weighted image.

Temporomandibular Disorder

Temporomandibular disorder is the second most common orofacial pain after tooth pain.[4] It is also the second most common chronic musculoskeletal condition after chronic low back pain.[16] **Table 3** provides a list of the most common TMJ-related disorders and the most appropriate imaging technique based on the updated recommendation from the panel of experts who developed the Diagnostic Criteria for Temporomandibular Disorders.[10] Imaging should not be obtained routinely, but should be based on the clinical needs of the patient. **Fig. 16** shows degenerative joint disease presentation in CBCT images.

TMJ inflammation and associated pain are reported to be commonly associated with juvenile idiopathic arthritis (JIA). Leksell and colleagues[17] reported on a case-control study of 41 patients with JIA and 41 age- and sex-matched healthy controls. TMJ pain was found to be prevalent in 33 out of 41 (80.5%) patients with JIA. In nearly a quarter of those patients, 9 out of 41 (22.0%), pain greatly affected their daily life. The alterations in bone metabolism and skeletal growth of JIA patients can cause open bite, mandibular retrusion, micrognathia, dental crowding, and facial asymmetry. The early detection of this condition and referral to an orthodontist or other specialist to reduce future occlusal and mandibular growth complications are essential for the management of pain and treatment.[18] **Fig. 17** illustrates CBCT presentations on a suspected JIA case.

Neuropathic Pain Disorders

Neuropathic pain is defined as pain caused by a lesion or disease affecting the somatosensory nervous system.[19] Because the trigeminal nerve is extensively distributed throughout the maxillofacial complex, it is commonly related to orofacial pain. Trigeminal neuropathy may result from lesions affecting all 5 segments of the trigeminal nerve: the brainstem segment, cisternal segment, Meckel cave, cavernous segment, and the peripheral segment. Dental procedures such as third molar extraction and dental implant placement[20–22] affect the peripheral segment of the trigeminal

Table 2
Intraoral pain disorders with selected imaging modalities and radiographic appearance

Common Pain Disorders	Selected Imaging Modality	Radiographic Appearance
Odontogenic pain		
Dental caries, fracture of crown or root	Intraoral/panoramic radiography	Radiolucent
Apical periodontitis	Intraoral/panoramic radiography/CBCT	Radiolucency at the apex of a tooth with caries or a large restoration, or radiopacity at the apex of a tooth with a large restoration
Periodontal pain (periodontal abscess)	Intraoral/panoramic radiography	Intercrestal and furcal bone loss
Pericoronitis	Cannot be diagnosed by radiograph alone, intraoral/panoramic radiography	A bony defect with sclerosing osteitis associated with the crown of an unerupted third molar
Pulpal and periodontal pain secondary to fractured teeth	Intraoral/panoramic radiography	Without displacement of tooth fragments, diagnosis is difficult
Odontogenic cyst or tumor	Depending on lesion size: intraoral/panoramic radiography/CBCT/CT	Radiolucent/radiopaque, displacement/resorption of teeth, expansion/perforation of cortical bone
Nonodontogenic pain		
Musculoskeletal, neurovascular, neuropathic, psychogenic	Panoramic radiography/CBCT/CT, MRI	Bone and soft tissue variations
Painful oral soft tissue lesions		
Localized mucogingival and glossal pain, infections, mucosal trauma, pain associated with cancer, geographic tongue, immune-mediated inflammatory conditions	Panoramic radiography/CBCT/CT to rule out osseous involvement	No radiographic evidence without osseous involvement

nerve and have the highest incidence of neuropathy. The incidence of altered sensation after implant placement has been found to range from 8.5% to 36%.[23] Other neuropathic orofacial pain can be related to root canal treatment and apicoectomy or may be found to be idiopathic. Trigeminal neuropathy does not occur in all patients who have nerve damage.

MRI may be used to image the trigeminal nerve itself.[19] However, damage in the peripheral segment can be evaluated using intraoral or panoramic radiography or CBCT/CT. Inadequate radiographic evaluation before a surgical procedure is the most common cause of trigeminal nerve damage.[24–26] Using CBCT/CT imaging before extraction or placement of dental implants to identify the relationship of the inferior alveolar canal to adjacent structures will help dental clinicians avoid surgical surprises (**Fig. 18**). In addition, it may be used in the detection of postsurgical

Table 3
Selected imaging modalities for the temporomandibular joint disorders

Common TMJ Disorders	Selected Imaging Modalities
Disc displacement	MRI in both open and closed position
Loose joint bodies (synovial chondromatosis)	Panoramic radiography/CBCT/CT, MRI
Inflammatory disturbances	
Degenerative joint disease	CBCT/CT
Rheumatoid arthritis	Panoramic radiography/CBCT/CT, MRI
Septic (infectious) arthritis	MRI, contrast-enhanced CT
Traumatic disturbances	
Fracture	Plain film/panoramic radiography/CBCT/CT, MRI
Dislocation	CBCT/CT, MRI
Ankylosis	CBCT/CT, MRI
Developmental disturbances	
Hyperplasia, hypoplasia, aplasia of the condyle and bifid condyle	Panoramic radiography/CBCT/CT

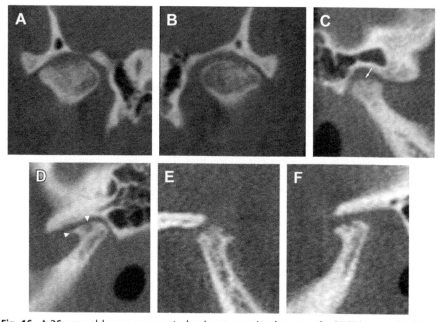

Fig. 16. A 36-year-old woman reported pain on opening her mouth. CBCT images (*A*, *B*) are corrected coronal views of the right and left condyles in the closed position, and (*C*, *D*) are corrected sagittal views of the right and left condyles in the closed position. Images (*E*, *F*) are corrected sagittal views of the right and left condyles in the open position. These images showed erosions of the right condyle (*arrow in C*) and osteophytes and subcortical pseudocysts (*arrowheads in D*) in the left condyle with translation to the articular eminence on both sides in maximum opening 32 mm.

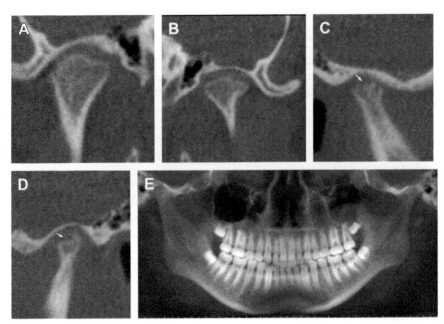

Fig. 17. A 13-year-old girl seeking orthodontic treatment complained of constant bilateral crepitus and spontaneous pain. CBCT images (*A, B*) are corrected coronal views, and (*C, D*) are corrected sagittal views of the right and left condyles in the closed position. These images showed the presence of erosions on the superior surfaces of both condyles (*arrows*). (*E*) A pseudopanoramic view shows asymmetry of mandibular ramus length. These findings are consistent with JIA.

nerve damage.[27–29] The American Academy of Oral and Maxillofacial Radiology recommends, "Cross-sectional imaging be used for the assessment of all dental implant sites and that CBCT is the imaging method of choice for gaining this information."[10] After an extensive literature search, including 176 published articles from January 1, 2000 to June 24, 2017, the American Academy of Periodontology Best Evidence Consensus Statement concluded that "Dental health care professionals should consider CBCT imaging when they expect the diagnostic information acquired will lead to better patient care, higher levels of safety, and improved clinical outcomes."[13]

Headache

The International Classification of Headache Disorders, 3rd edition (Beta version) has been published on the International Headache Society's Web site (https://www.ichd-3.org/classification-outline/). This classification may be found in **Table 4**.

Because headache is commonly associated with soft tissue and bony tissue of the head and neck, as indicated in **Table 4**, common imaging modalities for headache use nonenhanced or enhanced CT and T1- and T2-weighted MRI. In emergency situations, CT is the preferred diagnostic modality because of the shorter examination time, the ease of monitoring the patient, and the better patient access. If a vascular lesion is suspected, CT angiography may be performed. If an infectious lesion is suspected, MRI is a better choice than contrast-enhanced CT[30] to image an inflammatory process.

A

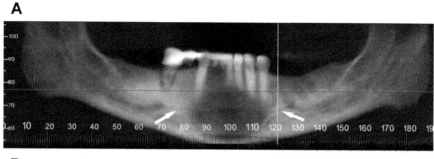

B

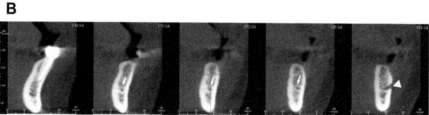

Fig. 18. Using CBCT imaging before placement of dental implants may be indicated to avoid surgical surprises and nerve damage. The patient shown has a prominent mandibular incisive canal (a continuation of the mandibular canal) bilaterally. (*A*) CBCT pseudopanoramic view and (*B*) left side cross-sectional images. Note the left mandibular incisive canal (*arrows*) and the mental foramen (*arrowhead*).

Table 4 International Headache Society classification	
Part 1: The primary headache	Migraine
	Tension-type headache
	Trigeminal autonomic cephalalgias
	Other primary headache disorders
Part 2: The secondary headache	Headache attributed to trauma or injury to the head and/or neck
	Headache attributed to cranial or cervical vascular disorder
	Headache attributed to nonvascular intracranial disorder
	Headache attributed to substance or its withdrawal
	Headache attributed to infection
	Headache attributed to disorder of homoeostasis
	Headache or facial pain attributed to disorder of the cranium, neck, eyes, ears, nose, sinuses, teeth, mouth, or other facial or cervical structure
	Headache attributed to psychiatric disorder
Part 3: Painful cranial neuropathies, other facial pains, and other headache	Painful lesions of the cranial nerves and other facial pains
	Other headache disorders

From International Headache Society. IHS classification outline. Available at: https://www.ichd-3.org/classification-outline/. Accessed November 30, 2017; with permission.

CT without intravenous contrast or CBCT is the primary modality for imaging the nasal cavity and paranasal sinuses.[31–33] CT/CBCT can delineate bony anatomic variants such as mucosal contact points between an osseous spur along a deviated nasal septum and the adjacent nasal turbinate that may predispose the patient to rhinogenic headache. CT/CBCT may also demonstrate all sources of infections and masses in the nasal cavity and paranasal sinuses. MRI complements CT/CBCT imaging by providing a better evaluation of infection and soft tissue mass, especially involving lesions in the brain or orbit. A recent study by Ohba and colleagues[34] reported on 86 patients with orofacial pain and 10 patients with paresthesia who had undergone 44 CT and 35 MRI examinations. They found 1 of 44 (2.3%) CT examinations detected lacunar infarction. In 35 patients who underwent MRI examinations, 13 (37.1%) were found to have pathosis such as trigeminal schwannoma and meningioma that resulted in neural compression of arteries. They indicated, "A high percentage of patients, who claimed orofacial pain and paresthesia, have other diseases in their brain, especially in elderly patients, and MRI is more useful than CT in evaluating these patients." A recent functional MRI study concluded that complex regional pain syndrome can be correlated with trigeminal neuropathy in the orofacial area.[35]

Other Sources of Orofacial Pain

Both dentists and physicians should be aware of pain associated with Eagle syndrome. A comprehensive review of this syndrome[36] recently reported the incidence of an elongated styloid process ranged from 4% to 7.3%. In cases of elongated styloid process, pain is one of the most common symptoms. Patients most often complained of unilateral pain on the side of the elongated styloid process. This pain may refer or radiate to the ear/jaw and present as otalgia or TMJ pain. Extraoral radiographs of the skull such as lateral cephalometric radiographs may be useful in demonstrating an elongated styloid process. Panoramic radiographs and CBCT/CT have been shown to be effective in diagnosing Eagle syndrome (**Fig. 19**). In a retrospective study[37] of 208 patients with orofacial pain who had CBCT performed for evaluation of the styloid process, 96 (46%) subjects had no elongation of the styloid process, 28 (13%) had left side elongation, 16 (8%) had right side elongation, and 68 (33%) had bilateral elongation of the styloid process. It was observed that patients suffering

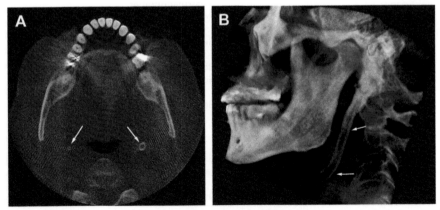

Fig. 19. (A) CBCT axial image and (B) left side 3-dimensional image show calcified elongated stylohyoid ligaments bilaterally (*arrows*), most prominently on the left side.

from orofacial pain, who also had an elongated styloid process, had an increased rate of neurologic complaints as compared with those who had no elongated styloid process. Symptoms of Eagle syndrome include dizziness, tinnitus, otalgia, dysphagia, foreign body sensation, and pain on turning head.[37] CT scans represent the gold standard for the diagnosis of elongated styloid process. CT scans add soft tissue data that allow for an appreciation of the relationship between the bony elongated styloid process and adjacent neurovascular structures.[38]

It is important to remember that the location or site of orofacial pain is not always related to the source of the pain. Therefore, finding the true source of the pain is paramount for both a diagnosis and an effective treatment.[6] For example, a nasopharyngeal carcinoma was found to masquerade as TMJ pain in a 50-year-old Caucasian woman for 3 months before being identified by CT and MRI studies.[39] Two cases of internal carotid artery dissection presented as maxillary tooth pain and was later identified by MRI and MR angiography.[40] A 59-year-old patient presented with a 4-year history of chronic oral pain and had 3 maxillary teeth extracted. Eventually MRI and CT angiography studies discovered that an internal carotid artery aneurysm that compressed the trigeminal nerve accounted for the pain felt within the distribution of the peripheral branches of the maxillary nerve.[41] Recently, Noma and colleagues[42] reported that a 77-year-old woman had unusual orofacial pain and headache associated with exfoliation glaucoma and conjunctivitis. Both panoramic radiograph and MRI showed no evidence of odontogenic lesion or intracranial/extracranial pathologic condition. These cases highlight the importance of a thorough knowledge of various causes of orofacial pain, the importance of advanced imaging studies, the value of consultation with or referral to appropriate medical/dental specialists, and interdisciplinary care for pain management.

SUMMARY

Imaging usefulness in the diagnosis of orofacial pain includes all modalities that cover the soft tissue and bony structures in the region of the head and neck. Imaging techniques may include either 2-dimensional and/or 3-dimensional imaging modalities. Each modality has its advantages and disadvantages. Both dentists and physicians should be aware of orofacial pain associated with a variety of sources and select the appropriate imaging technique based on the patient's medical and dental history and the clinical examination. Consideration of the radiation risk associated with each modality must be taken into consideration, but potential risk should not be at the expense of the anticipated gain in diagnostic information. The goal of imaging is to provide the clinician with information that will confirm or deny findings of the clinical examination and allow for the selection of an appropriate treatment.

REFERENCES

1. De Rossi SS. Orofacial pain: a primer. Dent Clin North Am 2013;57(3):383–92.
2. Haviv Y, Zini A, Etzioni Y, et al. The impact of chronic orofacial pain on daily life: the vulnerable patient and disruptive pain. Oral Surg Oral Med Oral Pathol Oral Radiol 2017;123(1):58–66.
3. Horst OV, Cunha-Cruz J, Zhou L, et al. Prevalence of pain in the orofacial regions in patients visiting general dentists in the Northwest Practice-based REsearch Collaborative in Evidence-based DENTistry research network. J Am Dent Assoc 2015;146(10):721–8.e3.

4. Oberoi SS, Hiremath SS, Yashoda R, et al. Prevalence of various orofacial pain symptoms and their overall impact on quality of life in a Tertiary Care Hospital in India. J Maxillofac Oral Surg 2014;13(4):533–8.

5. Sharav Y, Benoliel R. The diagnostic process. In: Huffman L, editor. Orofacial pain and headache. 2nd edition. Chicago: Quintessence Publishing Co, Inc; 2015. p. 1–29.

6. Leeuw RD, Klasser GD. General assessement of the orofacial pain patient and diagnostic classification of orofacial pain. In: de Leeuw R, Klasser GD, editors. Orofacial pain: guidelines for assessment, diagnosis, and management. 5th edition. Chicago: Quintessence Publishing Co, Inc; 2013. p. 25–57.

7. Rezaei F, Sharifi R, Shahrezaee HR, et al. Knowledge about chronic orofacial pain among general dentists of Kermanshah, Iran. Open Dent J 2017;11:221–9.

8. Schiffman E, Ohrbach R, Truelove E, et al. Diagnostic criteria for temporomandibular disorders (DC/TMD) for clinical and research applications: recommendations of the International RDC/TMD Consortium Network* and Orofacial Pain Special Interest Groupdagger. J Oral Facial Pain Headache 2014;28(1):6–27.

9. Mozzo P, Procacci C, Tacconi A, et al. A new volumetric CT machine for dental imaging based on the cone-beam technique: preliminary results. Eur Radiol 1998;8(9):1558–64.

10. Tyndall DA, Price JB, Tetradis S, et al. Position statement of the American Academy of Oral and Maxillofacial Radiology on selection criteria for the use of radiology in dental implantology with emphasis on cone beam computed tomography. Oral Surg Oral Med Oral Pathol Oral Radiol 2012;113(6):817–26.

11. AAE and AAOMR joint position statement: use of cone beam computed tomography in endodontics 2015 update. Oral Surg Oral Med Oral Pathol Oral Radiol 2015;120(4):508–12.

12. Patel S, Durack C, Abella F, et al. European Society of Endodontology position statement: the use of CBCT in endodontics. Int Endod J 2014;47(6):502–4.

13. Mandelaris GA, Scheyer ET, Evans M, et al. American Academy of Periodontology Best Evidence Consensus Statement on Selected Oral Applications for Cone-Beam Computed Tomography. J Periodontol 2017;88(10):939–45.

14. Horner K, O'Malley L, Taylor K, et al. Guidelines for clinical use of CBCT: a review. Dentomaxillofac Radiol 2015;44(1):20140225.

15. Scully C. Pain. In: Watt L, editor. Oral and maxillofacial medicine: the basis of diagnosis and treatment. London: Elsevier Health Sciences UK; 2012. p. 125–35.

16. Ahmad M, Schiffman EL. Temporomandibular joint disorders and orofacial pain. Dent Clin North Am 2016;60(1):105–24.

17. Leksell E, Ernberg M, Magnusson B, et al. Orofacial pain and dysfunction in children with juvenile idiopathic arthritis: a case-control study. Scand J Rheumatol 2012;41(5):375–8.

18. Carvalho RT, Braga FS, Brito F, et al. Temporomandibular joint alterations and their orofacial complications in patients with juvenile idiopathic arthritis. Rev Bras Reumatol 2012;52(6):907–11 [in English, Portuguese].

19. Graff-Radford S, Gordon R, Ganal J, et al. Trigeminal neuralgia and facial pain imaging. Curr Pain Headache Rep 2015;19(6):19.

20. Delcanho R, Moncada E. Persistent pain after dental implant placement: a case of implant-related nerve injury. J Am Dent Assoc 2014;145(12):1268–71.

21. Rodriguez-Lozano FJ, Sanchez-Perez A, Moya-Villaescusa MJ, et al. Neuropathic orofacial pain after dental implant placement: review of the literature and case report. Oral Surg Oral Med Oral Pathol Oral Radiol Endod 2010;109(4):e8–12.

22. Ardekian L, Dodson TB. Complications associated with the placement of dental implants. Oral Maxillofac Surg Clin North Am 2003;15(2):243–9.

23. Al-Sabbagh M, Okeson JP, Khalaf MW, et al. Persistent pain and neurosensory disturbance after dental implant surgery: pathophysiology, etiology, and diagnosis. Dent Clin North Am 2015;59(1):131–42.

24. Yilmaz Z, Ucer C, Scher E, et al. A survey of the opinion and experience of UK dentists: part 1: the incidence and cause of iatrogenic trigeminal nerve injuries related to dental implant surgery. Implant Dent 2016;25(5):638–45.

25. Yilmaz Z, Ucer C, Scher E, et al. A survey of the opinion and experience of UK dentists: part 2: risk assessment strategies and the management of iatrogenic trigeminal nerve injuries related to dental implant surgery. Implant Dent 2017;26(2): 256–62.

26. Ucer C, Yilmaz Z, Scher E, et al. A survey of the opinion and experience of UK dentists part 3: an evidence-based protocol of surgical risk management strategies in the mandible. Implant Dent 2017;26(4):532–40.

27. Al-Sabbagh M, Okeson JP, Bertoli E, et al. Persistent pain and neurosensory disturbance after dental implant surgery: prevention and treatment. Dent Clin North Am 2015;59(1):143–56.

28. Yepes JF, Al-Sabbagh M. Use of cone-beam computed tomography in early detection of implant failure. Dent Clin North Am 2015;59(1):41–56.

29. Steinberg MJ, Kelly PD. Implant-related nerve injuries. Dent Clin North Am 2015; 59(2):357–73.

30. Langner S, Kirsch M. Radiological diagnosis and differential diagnosis of headache. Rofo 2015;187(10):879–91.

31. Bricker A, Stultz T. Imaging for headache: what the neuroradiologist looks for. Otolaryngol Clin North Am 2014;47(2):197–219.

32. Pasha R, Soleja RQ, Ijaz MN. Imaging for headache: what the otolaryngologist looks for. Otolaryngol Clin North Am 2014;47(2):187–95.

33. Parks ET. Cone beam computed tomography for the nasal cavity and paranasal sinuses. Dent Clin North Am 2014;58(3):627–51.

34. Ohba S, Yoshimura H, Matsuda S, et al. Diagnostic role of magnetic resonance imaging in assessing orofacial pain and paresthesia. J Craniofac Surg 2014; 25(5):1748–51.

35. Lee YH, Lee KM, Kim HG, et al. Orofacial complex regional pain syndrome: pathophysiologic mechanisms and functional MRI. Oral Surg Oral Med Oral Pathol Oral Radiol 2017;124(2):e164–70.

36. Badhey A, Jategaonkar A, Anglin Kovacs AJ, et al. Eagle syndrome: a comprehensive review. Clin Neurol Neurosurg 2017;159:34–8.

37. Oztunc H, Evlice B, Tatli U, et al. Cone-beam computed tomographic evaluation of styloid process: a retrospective study of 208 patients with orofacial pain. Head Face Med 2014;10:5.

38. Murtagh RD, Caracciolo JT, Fernandez G. CT findings associated with Eagle syndrome. AJNR Am J Neuroradiol 2001;22(7):1401–2.

39. Khan J, Quek SY, Markman S. Nasopharyngeal carcinoma masquerading as TMJ orofacial pain. Quintessence Int 2010;41(5):387–9.

40. Abbott JJ, Newman AC, Schievink WI. Maxillary tooth pain as a symptom of internal carotid artery dissection: case series. J Am Dent Assoc 2017;148(6):399–403.

41. Stone SJ, Paleri V, Staines KS. Internal carotid artery aneurysm presenting as orofacial pain. J Laryngol Otol 2012;126(8):851–3.

42. Noma N, Iwasa M, Young A, et al. Orofacial pain and headaches associated with exfoliation glaucoma. J Am Dent Assoc 2017;148(12):936–40.

Musculoskeletal Disorders

Giovana Fernandes, DDS, MSc, PhD[a],*,
Daniela A.G. Gonçalves, DDS, MSc, PhD[a], Paulo Conti, DDS, MSc, PhD[b]

KEYWORDS

- Temporomandibular disorders • Multifactorial causalities • Myofascial pain
- Neuroplasticity • Degenerative joint disorders • Conservative treatments

KEY POINTS

- After rolling out dental pathologies, the most prevalent cause of a patient's chief orofacial complaint is musculoskeletal pain, usually referred to as temporomandibular disorder (TMD).
- The typical signs and symptoms of TMD are pain, limited range of motion, and temporomandibular joint sounds. Provocation and function, such as palpation and mastication, may aggravate the pain.
- TMD is a complex musculoskeletal disorder with a multifactorial etiology. The physical, behavioral, and emotional factors may overlap and interact resulting in the TMD signs and symptoms.
- Long-term peripheral inputs can produce changes in central structures related to pain processing. These adaptive changes are part of the central sensitization process that promotes amplification of the incoming signal, explaining the features of the centrally mediated pain.
- Management aims to reduce pain and to improve function with a combination of noninvasive therapies.

INTRODUCTION

Temporomandibular disorder (TMD), a type of musculoskeletal pain, is one of the main causes of painful conditions in the orofacial region. It is a condition that embraces some clinical problems involving the masticatory muscles, temporomandibular joints (TMJs), and associated structures. The most common signs and symptoms are pain, limited range of motion, and TMJ sounds.[1]

TMD is a highly prevalent condition. In a previous study, 39.2% of the sample reported at least one TMD symptom, and 25.6% of them reported some pain related

Disclosure Statement: The authors have nothing to disclose.
[a] Department of Dental Materials and Prosthodontics, Araraquara School of Dentistry, Univ Estadual Paulitsa, Humaitá, 1680 – Centro, Araraquara, São Paulo 14801-903, Brazil; [b] Department of Prosthodontics, Bauru School of Dentistry, University of São Paulo, Al Otavio P. Brisola 9-75, Bauru, São Paulo 17012-901, Brazil
* Corresponding author.
E-mail address: gfernandes@foar.unesp.br

to TMD.[2] The prevalence rate ranges between 4.0% and 25.5% in adolescents.[3–5] Among adults, an annual incidence rate of TMD diagnosis has been reported at 3.9%, and a rate of 4.6% for TMD pain is self-reported in adolescents.[6,7] It affects women more frequently than men with a sex ratio of approximately 2:1 (women:men) observed in population-based studies, and at least 4:1 in clinical settings.[8] There are no gender differences among children, but as the age increases, the sex ratio become approximately 2:1 (girls:boys) among young adults.[9]

It is relevant emphasizing that a single factor does not cause TMD. It results from the interaction of the risk factors. Therefore, the TMD etiology is multifactorial, with many predisposing, precipitating, or maintaining risk factors.[1] An extensive prospective study is being conducted to investigate the possible risk factors, assessing the genetic and phenotypic measures of biological, psychosocial, clinical, and health status characteristics.[10] Some of the investigated risk factors have been confirmed, but the study is also pointing for new findings, including biological factors, the role of endogenous opioid function, differences in genotypes, trauma, parafunction, and psychosocial factors.[11]

PATHOPHYSIOLOGY AND CLASSIFICATION OF ARTICULAR TEMPOROMANDIBULAR DISORDER

Articular TMD embraces several alterations affecting the hard and the soft tissues of the TMJ. The most recent and valid criteria classify the articular TMD in (1) joint pain, (2) joint disorders, (3) joint diseases, (4) fractures, and (5) congenital/developmental disorders (**Box 1**). Herein, we present the most common conditions.[1] A detailed description of the less common articular TMD is beyond the scope of this article, and readers are referred to reference publications.[1,12]

In general, the main signs and symptoms of articular TMD are pain in the joint area, limited and/or altered mandibular movement, and TMJ sounds such as clicking, popping, or crepitus.

Joint Pain

Arthralgia and arthritis are the 2 subtypes of joint pain. Arthralgia is affected by jaw movement, function, or parafunction, whereas arthritis, also called synovitis or capsulitis, is related to intra-articular inflammation or infection accompanied by edema, erythema, and/or increased temperature. In both cases, limitation of mandibular movement may occur due to the pain.[1,13] Evidence from human studies points to changes in the joint chemistry of patients with articular TMD, including, but not limited to, glutamate, cytokines, and serotonin (5-hydroxytryptamine [5-HT]). Overall, further investigations are needed to clarify the specific role of each of these mediators for diagnosis, treatment, and prognosis of joint conditions.[14]

Box 1
Temporomandibular joint disorder classification

1. Joint pain: arthralgia; arthritis

2. Joint disorders: disk disorders; other hypomobility disorders; hypermobility disorders

3. Joint diseases: degenerative joint disease; systemic arthritides; condylosis/idiopathic condylar resorption; osteochondritis dissecans; osteonecrosis; neoplasm; synovial chondromatosis

4. Fractures

5. Congenital/Developmental Disorders: aplasia; hypoplasia; hyperplasia

---

Joint Disorders: Disk Displacement

Disk disorders, a condition characterized by an abnormal relationship of the articular disk relative to the condyle is the most frequent condition affecting the TMJ.[1] The disks are usually displaced to the anterior and anteromedial position. Although they may be present, pain and mandibular movement alterations are not specifically related to disk displacement (DD). Its etiology is not totally clear, but includes alterations of the ligaments, intra-articular lubrication, and changes related to degenerative diseases.

The altered condyle-disk relationship in the closed mouth position can be reversible during mandibular movement (DD with reduction). Therefore, joint sounds (clicking, popping, or snapping noises) may occur during the opening and/or closing movements and indicate disk reduction. When the reduction does not occur, it is called DD without reduction. In both cases, movement limitation may be present and can be either intermittent (DD with reduction with intermittent locking), or persistent (DD without reduction with limited opening).[1,12]

The diagnostic criteria for DD without using TMJ imaging are not accurate enough. Therefore, a definitive diagnosis of DD for treatment decision-making in particular cases requires imaging.[12,15] Considering the necessity to evidence the disk (soft tissue) position, the TMJ MRI associated with a valid image criterion emerge as the best option.[12,16] Although DD is a highly prevalent condition,[17] most of the cases present a favorable prognosis, rarely requiring active treatment.[18] The primary options would be the conservative approaches focusing on reducing the pain and improving movements.[17,18]

Degenerative Joint Disease

The TMJ is a load-bearing joint with a significant and finite adaptive capacity to mechanical loading. Degenerative changes can develop progressively over time,[14,18] leading to a degradation of the articular cartilage, synovial inflammation, and alteration of the subchondral bone.[14,19] Its etiology is not fully understood, but some risk factors are overloading, age, systemic illness, and hormonal, nutritional, traumatic, mechanical, and genetic factors.[18–20] Some biochemical markers have been observed in the synovial fluid of TMJ, involving a complex cascade of events that result in soft and hard tissue degeneration.[14,19,20]

The principal clinical sign of degenerative joint disease (DJD) is TMJ sounds, especially crepitus, reflecting the degeneration of the articular cartilage and the subchondral bone, conferring an irregular aspect to the articular surfaces of the condyle and articular eminence, as well as the degeneration of the articular disk.[1,20] DJD may be secondary to systemic disorders or a local condition. Its diagnostic criteria include TMJ noise during jaw movement reported by the patient or detected in the clinical examination. A definitive diagnosis requires computed tomography imaging and should evidence the presence of subchondral cyst(s), erosion(s), generalized sclerosis, or osteophyte(s).[1,12,16]

PATHOPHYSIOLOGY OF MASTICATORY MUSCLE PAIN

Masticatory muscle pain is one of the most common manifestations of TMD, leading to facial pain of nonodontogenic origin.

Pain of muscular origin is generically classified as somatic, deep, and of musculoskeletal type. As somatic and profound, muscle pain usually requires a peripheral nociceptive stimulus to produce messages understood as pain in the central nervous system (CNS).[21] Muscle pain is diffuse, poorly localized by the patient, and clearly related to the muscle function; that is, the patient is able to report the initiation or exacerbation of pain when using the masticatory apparatus.

Tenderness to palpation and ability to elicit familiar pain that reproduces the pain felt by the patient during her or his activities is another important finding. This pressure has been suggested in the literature at approximately 1.5 to 1.8 kgf/cm^2.[22]

The most common clinical manifestations of masticatory muscle pain are localized myalgia and myofascial pain.[12] Localized myalgia refers to a condition in which the pain is felt in the past 30 days, is exacerbated by function, and the professional can reproduce the patient's complaint during the physical examination. In this case, the pain is restricted to the site of palpation. In the case of myofascial pain, the pain can spread beyond the site of palpation, but within the boundary of the muscle or referred to areas beyond the boundary of the muscle. Primary headaches, the presence of myofascial pain in the cervical region, and fibromyalgia are classic examples of overlapping diseases that can exacerbate masticatory muscle pain.[23]

Peripheral Sensitization of Muscle Nociceptors

The masticatory muscles are innervated by thinly myelinated and unmyelinated primary trigeminal afferent fibers with nonspecialized endings projecting to the trigeminal subnucleus caudalis (Group 3 [a-delta] and group 4 [c fibers]).[24,25] It has been suggested that after tissue damage, a cascade of peripheral events is triggered, leading to changes in the muscle environment. These changes are characterized by the release of neurovasoactive, algogenic substances (prostaglandin [PGE2], bradykinin, and histamine), followed by vasodilation and increased vascular permeability. Concurrently, these released substances sensitize peripheral nerve endings (mainly the PGE2), decreasing the primary afferent neuron threshold, starting the neural depolarization and eventually generating an action potential.[26] This increased activity of sensitized neurons is followed by the antidromic release of pain-related neuropeptides, especially substance P and calcitonin-related gene peptide (CGRP) in the muscle structure, increasing the inflammatory process, vasodilation, and venous congestion.[27] It has been known as neurogenic inflammation and is considered an essential step in the process of peripheral sensitization.

Central Sensitization of Second-Order Neurons

After entering the CNS, the peripheral nociceptive message is transmitted to second-order neurons, based on an electrical and chemical process. Substance P, CGRP, and glutamate seem to be relevant agents to transmit the message to the trigeminal subnucleus caudalis neurons.

After a prolonged or significant peripheral tissue stimulation, receptors such as N-methyl D-aspartate, initially blocked by the Mg^{++} in a short-lasting stimulus situation, become extremely active, triggering a cascade of intracellular events inside the second-order neuron, involving Ca^{++} influx, phosphorylation, and gene expression. The result of these alterations is a hyperexcited neuron, which starts to produce nitric oxide, released in the synaptic cleft, increasing the sensitization process.[28]

These phenomena are known as central sensitization, and now a nonpainful, innocuous stimulus is interpreted as a painful event.[29] Central sensitization has been considered a crucial event in the persistent muscle pain scenario, which makes the pain become independent of any peripheral stimuli to occur or to be overinterpreted at the central level. The clinical result of these changes is the secondary hyperalgesia; that is, exacerbated response to a regular nociceptive stimulus.

Impaired Antinociceptive Descending System

In a typical situation, when nociceptive information arrives from the periphery and reaches the CNS at the spinal cord level, a sequence of descending stimuli is triggered to filter such information. In other words, the original nociceptive information is exacerbated or attenuated by a complex combination of different neurotransmitters.[30]

Several areas, such as the periaqueductal gray matter, nucleus raphe magnus (NRM), lateral nuclei of the reticular formation, and locus coeruleus, are directly involved in synthesizing and releasing descending substances that will modulate the ascending information.

The inhibition of the trigeminothalamic neurons at the trigeminal subnucleus caudalis level is based on the initial activity of the transmitter serotonin (5-HT), released by fibers from the NRM. This descending activation stimulates the activity of the neurotransmitter enkephalin and gamma-aminobutyric acid, which eventually interferes with the release of excitatory neurotransmitters, decreasing the firing of second-order neurons, and partially inhibiting the pain information transmission.[31]

In many pathologic conditions, like fibromyalgia, chronic tension-type headache, and myofascial pain, this system is somehow impaired, allowing the peripheral stimuli to reach central centers with only partial (or total absence) filtering.[32]

EVIDENCE-BASED TREATMENT MODALITIES

Because of the TMD multifactorial etiology and variety of clinical presentations, the treatment options for this disorder are diverse. As described previously, pain is one of the most frequent TMD complaints, and there is an already well-established consensus that most painful TMD cases respond well to the conservative and reversible therapies.[1] It has been demonstrated that these therapies can reduce pain and improve function. Therefore, the reversible approaches are indicated as the first option in TMD management.[1] Based on current evidence, the most common reversible and conservative treatments for TMD (**Table 1**) are discussed.

Education and Self-Management

Education and self-management therapy is considered the first approach for the treatment of TMD and is highly effective independent of additional interventions that can be used.[34] The educational approach aims to explain the nature, etiology, and prognosis of the condition, including the notion that parafunctional activity and psychosocial factors play a role in the pathogenesis of musculoskeletal pain.[44] Previous investigations comparing education with other treatment modalities showed that increasing the patients' responsibilities and addressing the psychosocial factors could yield better results.[45] Likewise, the use of home physical therapy added to education also has been indicated, because it can be efficacious for patients with TMD pain.[46] Home physical therapy includes exercises, relaxation techniques with diaphragmatic breathing, automassage of the masticatory muscles, application of moist heat, and stretching and coordination exercises, such as proprioceptive training and posture.

Electrophysiological Therapy

Low-level laser therapy (LLLT) is a safe, affordable, and nonpharmacological therapeutic modality in TMD treatment. However, it is relevant to emphasize that there is no consensus in the scientific literature about the doses and protocols of LLLT, and this could complicate its effective use in clinical practice. The best current evidence about its efficacy indicates that this therapy is limited in reducing pain in patients with TMD, but promotes significant improvement in the functional aspects involving jaw mobility, such as mouth opening and chewing.[36] In the myofascial trigger point area, laser therapy helps to break the vicious cycle of pain, muscle spasm, and further pain.[35]

Table 1
The main temporomandibular disorder treatment modalities

Treatment Modality	Main Effects
Education	• Reduction of the strain of the masticatory system • Relaxation • Reduction of muscle activity[33]
Home physical therapy	• Musculoskeletal pain relief • Reduction of inflammation • Improvement of muscle coordination • Regeneration of soft tissues[34]
Low-lever laser	• Analgesic/anti-inflammatory effects • Tissue regeneration • Inactivation of myofascial trigger points[35,36]
Ultrasound	• Reduction of inflammation • Muscle relaxation • Increase the blood flow[37]
Transcutaneous electrical nerve stimulation	• Increase the activity of descending pain modulation system[38]
Dry needling	• Promote peripheral healing • Stimulate endogenous modulation[39]
Botox	• Temporarily decrease muscle contraction • Control peripheral sensitization[40]
Nonsteroidal anti-inflammatory drugs	• Reduction of joint pain and inflammation[20]
Cyclobenzaprine/Tizanidine	• Promote muscle relaxation associated with an antinociceptive effect[41]
Tricyclic antidepressants	• Pain control by increasing the levels of serotonin and/or noradrenaline[42]
Occlusal Splint	• Decrease muscle overload • Stimulate cognitive awareness[43]

There are few and controversial pieces of evidence regarding the effect of ultrasound therapy on TMD pain and dysfunction. Some evidence indicates that ultrasound therapy was not effective when used alone in relieving symptoms; however, it is more efficient when used as an adjunct to the other modalities of therapy.[47]

Finally, the use of the transcutaneous electrical nerve stimulation (TENS) in TMD pain management could be controversial. The lack of clear protocols for TMD could explain such differences, considering variations in the stimulation frequency and total time application of TENS. The protocol that seems to be more favorable for the treatment of TMD pain consists in total time application of 50 minutes using variations of low and high frequency, with a sweep of 4 Hz (first 25 minutes) and 100 Hz (last 25 minutes) due to a complementary analgesic mechanism when adopting high and low frequencies.[38]

Needling and Botulin Toxin

Needling techniques can be divided into injection techniques, often referred to as "wet needling," which use hollow-bore needles to deliver corticosteroids, anesthetics, sclerosants, botulinum toxins, or other agents,[48] and dry needling (DN), which refers to the insertion of thin monofilament needles, as used in the practice of acupuncture, without the use of injectate.[49]

The advantages of DN are increasingly documented,[50] and include an immediate reduction in local, referred, and widespread pain, restoration of range of motion, muscle activation patterns,[51] and a normalization of the immediate chemical environment of active myofascial trigger points. Moreover, there is evidence that DN can reduce peripheral and central sensitization.[48] Jung and colleagues[52] published a systematic review of 7 randomized controlled trials and found only limited evidence for the use of acupuncture for the symptomatic treatment of TMD.

Botulinum toxin type A (BoNT-A) is rising as the most popular therapy within injection techniques used to control myofascial pain. This pro-toxin polypeptide is the fermentation product of Clostridium botulinum, a gram-positive anaerobic bacteria in spore forming.[40] Due to its high affinity for cholinergic synapses, the canonical effect of BoNT-A (and of the other serotypes) is mainly exerted as a selective inhibitor of evoked acetylcholine release from cholinergic nerve endings at the skeletal neuromuscular junction, causing a reversible muscle relaxation in therapeutic dosages.[53]

At the beginning of the use of BoNT-A for the treatment of muscular spasticity, it was observed that pain associated with muscle spasms was significantly attenuated to the degree that exceeded what would be anticipated from the simple reduction of muscle contraction.[54] Currently, preclinical models show that local injections of BoNT/A1 or BoNT/B1 have profound effects on various pain states and that it inhibits the release of various nociceptive mediators, such as substance P, the peptide related to the calcitonin gene, and glutamate.[55] Consequently, the clinical applications of BoNT-A to control various types of chronic orofacial pain (TMD, secondary headache, and neuralgias) are promising, but the few randomized, double-blind, placebo, clinical studies in the literature present conflicting results regarding the efficacy of this treatment for these disorders.[56]

Furthermore, there is no evidence in which specific mechanisms of chronic pain or in which somatosensory profiles BoNT-A acts to control pain.[57] No differences were reported when comparing DN and BoNT-A for myofascial pain[58] indicating that due to its high cost, BoNT-A should be reserved for refractory cases, in which the expected effects could not be achieved with conservative treatments.

Pharmacotherapy

The pharmacotherapy for TMD, in most cases, will only provide an improvement of symptoms and must be administered simultaneously with other therapeutic modalities. Unfortunately, the current pharmacologic treatment for TMD is largely empirical, because there is a lack of scientific evidence that demonstrates the efficacy of the various drugs.

Considering joint inflammation, it seems reasonable that nonsteroidal anti-inflammatory drugs, which are both analgesic and anti-inflammatory, would be the drug of choice for this TMJ pain (arthralgia or arthritis/arthrosis). However, the efficacy of this class of drug has been limited to just a few agents, because naproxen showed a significant reduction in pain when compared with celecoxib and placebo,[59] and a significantly greater effect of diclofenac compared with placebo was not found.[60]

Cyclobenzaprine is commonly used for TMD muscle pain.[61] A systematic review supports evidence for the efficacy of cyclobenzaprine, albeit with a fairly short follow-up time of 3 weeks.[62] Tizanidine also acts as a central muscle relaxant, producing muscular relaxation associated with an antinociceptive effect, although lesser than cyclobenzaprine.[41]

For patients with chronic TMD, presenting alteration in central pain processing, some drug agents with CNS activity can be indicated. Among them, the tricyclic antidepressants (eg, amitriptyline) are most commonly used. According to some investigators, the use of tricyclic antidepressants in patients with TMD pain seems to be effective in the control of pain.[42]

Occlusal Splint

Occlusal splints are one the most used treatment modalities for the management of TMD, especially those from the masticatory muscles, for more than 100 years. The rigid resin acrylic, full-coverage, canine-guided, stabilization occlusal splint is doubtless the most used and studied. Systematic reviews[63,64] concluded that stabilization splints are beneficial for reducing pain in patients with masticatory muscle myalgia when compared with no treatment. It has been believed that different peripheral, central, and behavioral alterations take place when a splint is used. Diminution in muscle activity, improvement in dental occlusal, with the incorporation of "ideal occlusal" features, increase in the vertical dimension of occlusion, cognitive alterations, and the placebo effect[65] are described as potential positive effects of occlusal splints.[66]

The decrease in the strain to the masticatory system, accompanied by a positive impact of the patient's initial reaction to a professional orientation, is also important for the reduction in pain levels.[67] The favorable natural course and the self-limiting evolution of TMD pain,[68,69] associated with the regression toward the mean phenomenon,[70] may also play a role in this scenario. A positive effect of the use of occlusal splints in many psychological aspects in subjects with a chief complaint of masticatory myofascial pain has also been demonstrated in a recent publication.[71]

It has also been reported that intraoral appliances have a marked "cognitive awareness concept," associated with the presence of a strange object (the appliance) inside the mouth, warning about the potentially harmful use of the jaw, which could lead to temporary[43] alterations in the intramuscular recruitment pattern.

SUMMARY

To summarize, TMD is a complex musculoskeletal disorder with multifactorial etiology, in which physical, behavioral, and emotional factors overlap and interact among them. Therefore, a multimodality conservative approach must be recommended, based on an accurate diagnosis.

REFERENCES

1. The American Academy of Orofacial Pain. In: de Leeuw R, Klasser G, editors. Orofacial pain: guidelines for assessment, diagnosis, and management. 5th edition. New York: Quintessence Publishing Co; 2013. p. 312.
2. Gonçalves DADG, Dal Fabbro AL, Campos JADB, et al. Symptoms of temporomandibular disorders in the population: an epidemiological study. J Orofac Pain 2010;24(3):270–8.
3. Drangsholt M, LeResche L. Temporomandibular disorders pain. In: Crombie I, Croft P, Linton S, et al, editors. Epidemiology of pain. 1st edition. Seattle (WA): IASP Press; 1999. p. 321.
4. Nilsson I-M, List T, Drangsholt M. Prevalence of temporomandibular pain and subsequent dental treatment in Swedish adolescents. J Orofac Pain 2005; 19(2):144–50.
5. Fernandes G, van Selms MKA, Gonçalves DAG, et al. Factors associated with temporomandibular disorders pain in adolescents. J Oral Rehabil 2015;42(2):113–9.
6. Nilsson I-M, List T, Drangsholt M. Incidence and temporal patterns of temporomandibular disorder pain among Swedish adolescents. J Orofac Pain 2007; 21(2):127–32.

7. Slade GD, Bair E, Greenspan JD, et al. Signs and symptoms of first-onset TMD and sociodemographic predictors of its development: the OPPERA prospective cohort study. J Pain 2013;14(12):T20–32.

8. LeResche L. Epidemiology of temporomandibular disorders: implications for the investigation of etiologic factors. Crit Rev Oral Biol Med 1997;8(3):291–305.

9. LeResche L, Mancl LA, Drangsholt MT, et al. Predictors of onset of facial pain and temporomandibular disorders in early adolescence. Pain 2007;129(3):269–78.

10. Maixner W, Diatchenko L, Dubner R, et al. Orofacial pain prospective evaluation and risk assessment study–the OPPERA study. J Pain 2011;12(11 Suppl):T4–11.

11. Slade GD, Ohrbach R, Greenspan JD, et al. Painful temporomandibular disorder: decade of discovery from OPPERA studies. J Dent Res 2016;95(10):1084–92.

12. Schiffman E, Ohrbach R, Truelove E, et al. Diagnostic criteria for temporomandibular disorders (DC/TMD) for clinical and research applications: recommendations of the International RDC/TMD Consortium Network* and Orofacial Pain Special Interest Group†. J Oral Facial Pain Headache 2014;28(1):6–27.

13. Alstergren P, Kopp S. Pain and synovial fluid concentration of serotonin in arthritic temporomandibular joints. Pain 1997;72(1–2):137–43.

14. Ernberg M. The role of molecular pain biomarkers in temporomandibular joint internal derangement. J Oral Rehabil 2017;44(6):481–91.

15. Schiffman E, Ohrbach R. Executive summary of the diagnostic criteria for temporomandibular disorders for clinical and research applications. J Am Dent Assoc 2016;147(6):438–45.

16. Hatcher DC. Imaging of the TMJ and associated structures. In: Greene CS, Laskin DM, editors. Treatment of TMDs: bridging the gap between advances in research and clinical patient management. 1st edition. Hanover Park (IL): Quintessence Publishing Co, Inc; 2013. p. 204.

17. Naeije M, te Veldhuis AH, te Veldhuis EC, et al. Disc displacement within the human temporomandibular joint: a systematic review of a "noisy annoyance." J Oral Rehabil 2013;40(2):139–58.

18. Al-Baghdadi M, Durham J, Steele J. Timing interventions in relation to temporomandibular joint closed lock duration: a systematic review of "locking duration." J Oral Rehabil 2014;41(1):24–58.

19. Emshoff R. Pathophysiology of intracapsular inflammation and degeneration. In: Greene CS, Laskin DM, editors. Treatment of TMDs: bridging the gap between advances in research and clinical patient management. 1st edition. Hanover Park (IL): Quintessence Publishing Co, Inc; 2013. p. 204.

20. Tanaka E, Detamore MS, Mercuri LG. Degenerative disorders of the temporomandibular joint: etiology, diagnosis, and treatment. J Dent Res 2008;87(4):296–307.

21. Mense S. Peripheral mechanisms of muscle pain: response behavior of muscle nociceptors and factors eliciting local muscle pain. In: Mense S, Gerwin RD, editors. Muscle pain: understanding the mechanisms. Springer; 2010. p. 50–8.

22. Santos Silva RS, Conti PCR, Lauris JRP, et al. Pressure pain threshold in the detection of masticatory myofascial pain: an algometer-based study. J Orofac Pain 2005;19(4):318–24.

23. Costa YM, Conti PCR, de Faria FA, et al. Temporomandibular disorders and painful comorbidities: clinical association and underlying mechanisms. Oral Surg Oral Med Oral Pathol Oral Radiol Endod 2017;123(3):288–97.

24. Coutaux A, Adam F, Willer J-C, et al. Hyperalgesia and allodynia: peripheral mechanisms. Joint Bone Spine 2005;72(5):359–71.

25. Mense S. Algesic agents exciting muscle nociceptors. Exp Brain Res 2009; 196(1):89–100.

26. Mense S. The pathogenesis of muscle pain. Curr Pain Headache Rep 2003;7(6):
    419–25.
27. Marchand F, Perretti M, McMahon SB. Role of the immune system in chronic pain.
    Nat Rev Neurosci 2005;6(7):521–32.
28. Hoheisel U, Unger T, Mense S. A block of spinal nitric oxide synthesis leads to
    increased background activity predominantly in nociceptive dorsal horn neuro-
    nes in the rat. Pain 2000;88(3):249–57.
29. Woolf CJ. Central sensitization: implications for the diagnosis and treatment of
    pain. Pain 2011;152(Supplement):S2–15.
30. Basbaum AI, Fields HL. Endogenous pain control systems: brainstem spinal
    pathways and endorphin circuitry. Annu Rev Neurosci 1984;7(1):309–38.
31. Vanegas H, Schaible H-G. Descending control of persistent pain: inhibitory or
    facilitatory? Brain Res Brain Res Rev 2004;46(3):295–309.
32. Hilgenberg-Sydney PB, Kowacs PA, Conti PCR. Somatosensory evaluation in
    dysfunctional syndrome patients. J Oral Rehabil 2016;43(2):89–95.
33. Glaros AG, Forbes M, Shanker J, et al. Effect of parafunctional clenching on
    temporomandibular disorder pain and proprioceptive awareness. Cranio 2000;
    18(3):198–204. Available at: http://www.ncbi.nlm.nih.gov/pubmed/11202838.
34. Story WP, Durham J, Al-Baghdadi M, et al. Self-management in temporomandib-
    ular disorders: a systematic review of behavioural components. J Oral Rehabil
    2016;43(10):759–70.
35. Uemoto L, Nascimento de Azevedo R, Almeida Alfaya T, et al. Myofascial trigger
    point therapy: laser therapy and dry needling. Curr Pain Headache Rep 2013;
    17(9):357.
36. Chen J, Huang Z, Ge M, et al. Efficacy of low-level laser therapy in the treatment
    of TMDs: a meta-analysis of 14 randomised controlled trials. J Oral Rehabil 2015;
    42(4):291–9.
37. Rai S, Goel S, Singh S, et al. Prospective utility of therapeutic ultrasound in
    dentistry—review with recent comprehensive update. Adv Biomed Res 2012;
    1(1):47.
38. Vance CGT, Dailey DL, Rakel BA, et al. Using TENS for pain control: the state of
    the evidence. Pain Manag 2014;4(3):197–209.
39. Fernández-Carnero J, La Touche R, Ortega-Santiago R, et al. Short-term effects
    of dry needling of active myofascial trigger points in the masseter muscle in pa-
    tients with temporomandibular disorders. J Orofac Pain 2010;24:106–12.
40. Wheeler A, Smith H. Botulinum toxins: mechanisms of action, antinociception and
    clinical applications. Toxicology 2013;306:124–46.
41. Alencar FG Jr, Viana PG, Zamperini C, et al. Patient education and self-care for
    the management of jaw pain upon awakening: a randomized controlled clinical
    trial comparing the effectiveness of adding pharmacologic treatment with cyclo-
    benzaprine or tizanidine. J Oral Facial Pain Headache 2014;28(2):119–27.
42. Plesh O, Curtis D, Levine J, et al. Amitriptyline treatment of chronic pain in pa-
    tients with temporomandibular disorders. J Oral Rehabil 2000;27:834–41.
43. Jokstad A, Mo A, Krogstad B. Clinical comparison between two different splint designs
    for temporomandibular disorder therapy. Acta Odontol Scand 2005;63:218–26.
44. Haldorsen EM, Kronholm K, Skouen JS, et al. Multimodal cognitive behavioral
    treatment of patients sicklisted for musculoskeletal pain: a randomized controlled
    study. Scand J Rheumatol 1998;27(1):16–25.
45. Kotiranta U, Suvinen T, Forssell H. Tailored treatments in temporomandibular dis-
    orders: where are we now? A systematic qualitative literature review. J Oral Facial
    Pain Headache 2014;28(1):28–37.

46. Michelotti A, Steenks MH, Farella M, et al. The additional value of a home physical therapy regimen versus patient education only for the treatment of myofascial pain of the jaw muscles: short-term results of a randomized clinical trial. J Orofac Pain 2004;18(2):114–25.
47. Ucar M, Sarp Ü, Koca İ, et al. Effectiveness of a home exercise program in combination with ultrasound therapy for temporomandibular joint disorders. J Phys Ther Sci 2014;26(12):1847–9.
48. Dommerholt J. Dry needling—peripheral and central considerations. J Man Manip Ther 2011;19(4):223–7.
49. Casanueva B, Rivas P, Rodero B, et al. Short-term improvement following dry needle stimulation of tender points in fibromyalgia. Rheumatol Int 2015;34(6):861–6.
50. Dommerholt J, Gerwin RD. Neurophysiological effects of trigger point needling therapies. In: Fernández de las Peñas C, Arendt-Nielsen L, Gerwin RD, editors. Diagnosis and management of tension type and cervicogenic headache. Boston (MA): Jones & Bartlett; 2010. p. 247–59.
51. Lucas K, Rich P, Polus B. Muscle activation patterns in the scapular positioning muscles during loaded scapular plane elevation: the effects of latent myofascial trigger points. Clin Biomech 2010;21:765–70.
52. Jung A, Shin B, Lee M, et al. Acupuncture for treating temporomandibular joint disorders: a systematic review and meta-analysis of randomized, sham-controlled trials. J Dent 2011;39(5):341–50.
53. Matak I, Lacković Z. Botulinum toxin A, brain and pain. Prog Neurobiol 2014;120: 39–59.
54. Brin M, Fahn S, Moskowitz C, et al. Localized injections of botulinum toxin for the treatment of focal dystonia and hemifacial spasm. Mov Disord 1987;2(4): 237–54.
55. Glaros AG, Kim-Weroha N, Lausten L, et al. Comparison of habit reversal and a behaviorally-modified dental treatment for temporomandibular disorders: a pilot investigation. Appl Psychophysiol Biofeedback 2007;32(3–4):149–54.
56. Ernberg M, Hedenberg-Magnusson B, List T, et al. Efficacy of botulinum toxin type A for treatment of persistent myofascial TMD pain: a randomized, controlled, double-blind multicenter study. Pain 2011;152:1988–96.
57. Pellett S, Tepp W, Whitemarsh R, et al. In vivo onset and duration of action varies for botulinum neurotoxin A subtypes 1-5. Toxicon 2015;107(Pt A):37–42.
58. Kamanli A, Kaya A, Ardicoglu O, et al. Comparison of lidocaine injection, botulinum toxin injection, and dry needling to trigger points in myofascial pain syndrome. Rheumatol Int 2005;25(8):604–11.
59. Ta LE, Dionne RA. Treatment of painful temporomandibular joints with a cyclooxygenase-2 inhibitor: a randomized placebo-controlled comparison of celecoxib to naproxen. Pain 2004;111(1):13–21.
60. Ekberg E. Treatment of temporomandibular disorders of arthrogeneous origin. Controlled double-blind studies of a non-steroidal anti-inflammatory drug and a stabilisation appliance. Swed Dent J Suppl 1998;131:1–57.
61. Denucci DJ, Dionne RA, Dubner R. Identifying a neurobiologic basis for drug therapy in TMDs. J Am Dent Assoc 1996;127(5):581–93.
62. Häggman-Henrikson B, Alstergren P, Davidson T, et al. Pharmacological treatment of oro-facial pain—health technology assessment including a systematic review with network meta-analysis. J Oral Rehabil 2017;44(10): 800–26.
63. Chao Z, Jun-Yi W, Dong-Lai D, et al. Efficacy of splint therapy for the management of temporomandibular disorders. Oncotarget 2016;7(51):84043–53.

64. Kuzmanovic P, Dodic S, Lazic V, et al. Occlusal stabilization splint for patients with temporomandibular disorders: meta-analysis of short and long term effects. PLoS One 2017;12(2):e0171296.

65. Greene C, Goddard G, Macaluso G, et al. Topical review: placebo responses and therapeutic responses. How are they related? J Orofac Pain 2009;23:93–107.

66. Conti P, de Alencar E, da Mota Corrêa A, et al. Behavioural changes and occlusal splints are effective in the management of masticatory myofascial pain: a short-term evaluation. J Oral Rehabil 2012;39(10):754–60.

67. Dube C, Rompre P, Manzini C, et al. Quantitative polygraphic controlled study on efficacy and safety of oral splint devices in tooth-grinding subjects. J Dent Res 2004;83:398–403.

68. Carlsson G. Some dogmas related to prosthodontics, temporomandibular disorders and occlusion. Acta Odontol Scand 2010;68(6):313–22.

69. Alencar FJ, Becker A. Evaluation of different occlusal splints and counselling in the management of myofascial pain dysfunction. J Oral Rehabil 2009;36:79–85.

70. Whitney C, Von Korff M. Regression to the mean in treated versus untreated chronic pain. Pain 1992;50:281–5.

71. Costa Y, Porporatti A, Stuginski-Barbosa J, et al. Additional effect of occlusal splints on the improvement of psychological aspects in temporomandibular disorder subjects: a randomized controlled trial. Arch Oral Biol 2015;60(5):738–44.

Neuropathic Orofacial Pain

Janina Christoforou, DClinDent(OralMed/OralPath), FRACDS(GDP),
MRACDS(OralMed), FOMAA

KEYWORDS

- Neuralgia • Facial pain • Neuritis • Herpes zoster

KEY POINTS

- Neuropathic orofacial pain is described as a pain caused by a lesion or disease of the somatosensory nervous system.
- Nociceptive stimuli in the orofacial region is modulated as it ascends to the thalamus and then to the somatosensory areas of the cortex.
- Complexities in individual pain perceptions are due to the influence of cognitive, affective, and motivational factors.
- Research continues to be undertaken to introduce more effective management options for neuropathic orofacial pain patients.

INTRODUCTION

Neuropathic orofacial pain is described as a pain caused by a lesion or disease of the somatosensory nervous system. Nociceptive stimuli in the orofacial region move along the trigeminal pathway, being modulated as it ascends to the thalamus. It is at this point where pain is perceived and then projected to the somatosensory areas of the cerebral cortex, allowing interpretation of this stimulus. Further complexities in individual pain perceptions are due to the influence of a myriad of cognitive, behavioral, affective, and motivational factors.

Neuropathic pain is broadly separated into episodic and continuous pain (**Fig. 1**).

TRIGEMINAL NEURALGIA

Trigeminal neuralgia (TN) is a paroxysmal, unilateral, short-lasting facial pain. Onset of TN may be abrupt or through a rarer preceding syndrome termed *pre-TN*.

Pretrigeminal Neuralgia

Pretrigeminal neuralgia (PTN) may precede TN in 18% of patients.[1] PTN is characterized by

Disclosure Statement: The author has nothing to disclose.
University of Western Australia, School of Dentistry, 17 Monash Avenue, Nedlands, Western Australia 6009, Australia
E-mail address: janinachristoforou@gmail.com

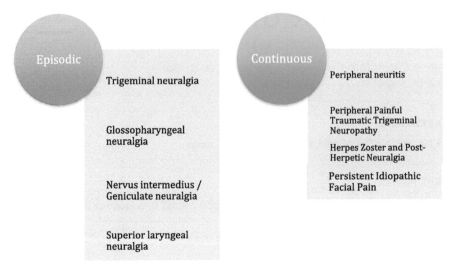

Fig. 1. Types of neuropathic pain in the orofacial region.

- A dull, continuous pain in one of the jaws that lasts from days to years before becoming typical.

The lack of clear and consistent diagnostic criteria makes this a problematic entity to recognize; it is usually diagnosed when all other possibilities are exhausted or in retrospect when classical TN develops.

Two subsets of TN are recognized (**Fig. 2**).

Atypical Trigeminal Neuralgia

Atypical trigeminal neuralgias are cases that present with most but not all diagnostic criteria and are not recognized by any current classification. Features of atypical cases may include the following:

- A low-grade background pain
- Longer-lasting attacks
- Increased resistance to therapy
- A higher rate of recurrence[4]

Clinical Presentation

- Sharp, short-lasting pain
- Usually unilateral
- The presence of trigger zones
  - Innocuous stimuli in these areas, which lead to pain
- Triggering stimuli include talking, chewing, touch, temperature, wind, and shaving
  - However, triggers are not always present or identifiable[5]

Diagnosis

The diagnosis of TN is based on a thorough clinical examination and patient history. Imaging such as MRI and MR angiography is necessary to investigate possible vascular impingement and exclude intracranial pathosis.

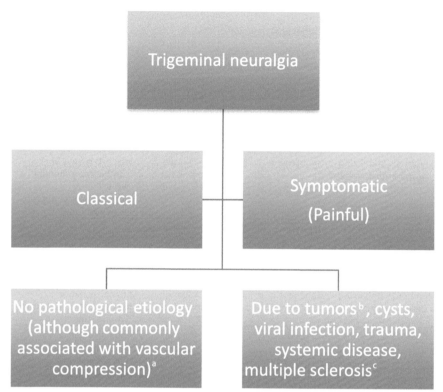

Fig. 2. Subsets of TN. [a] Commonly involving the superior cerebellar artery. [b] Middle and posterior cranial fossa tumors, cerebellopontine angle tumors, meningiomas.[2] [c] Clinically predictive of multiple sclerosis are bilateral pain (14%) and young age.[3]

Pathogenesis

The peripheral nerve morphologic changes occurring in both classical and symptomatic TN lead to structural changes, such as focal demyelination and afferent hyperexcitability and ectopic firing.[6]

Central nervous system neuroplasticity occurs in the presence of these changes and will affect the clinical phenotype and response to therapy.[7]

Management

Pharmacologic management is the first-line therapy for TN (**Table 1**):

1. Initiation of carbamazepine
   a. If there are side effects
      i. Reduce the dose of carbamazepine and add baclofen
      ii. Or trial oxcarbazepine
   b. In resistant cases or when carbamazepine is contraindicated
      i. Gabapentin or pregabalin
   c. In refractory cases
      i. Add-on therapy with lamotrigine or baclofen should be trialed before changing drugs[7]

Table 1
Pharmacologic agents for trigeminal neuralgia

Class	Medication	Dosage	Efficacy
Membrane stabilizing drugs: anticonvulsant	Carbamazepine	Started at 300 mg and maintenance at 800–1600 mg/d[8]	Effectiveness reduces over time
Membrane stabilizing drugs: anticonvulsant	Oxcarbazepine	Started at 600 mg/d and maintenance at 1200–1800 mg/d[8]	May have similar efficacy to carbamazepine[9] but decreases its effectiveness over time[9]
Membrane stabilizing drugs: anticonvulsant	Lamotrigine	Started at 25 mg/d and maintenance at 200–400 mg/d[8]	More often used in combination therapy with carbamazepine but also as monotherapy[10]
Central nervous system depressant	Baclofen	Started at 15 mg/d and maintenance at 60–80 mg/d[8]	More often used in combination therapy with other medication, that is, carbamazepine[11]
Membrane stabilizing drugs: anticonvulsant	Gabapentin	Started at 150 mg and maintenance at 300–900 mg/d[12]	Minimal evidence Effective first- and second-line treatment[12]
Membrane stabilizing drugs: anticonvulsant	Pregabalin	Started at 150 mg and maintenance at 150–600 mg/d[13]	Minimal evidence Effectiveness in treatment has been shown[13]
Membrane stabilizing drugs: anticonvulsant	Topiramate	Started at 25 mg bid and maintenance at 100 mg bid[14]	Effective in TN secondary to multiple sclerosis[14]
Triptan-selective serotonin receptor agonist	Sumatriptan	3 mg subcutaneously[15]	Success in refractory TN[15]
Neurotoxin	Botulinum toxin A	25–75 units transcutaneously (7.5 units per injection site)[17]	Some success in refractory cases[16] Insufficient scientific evidence

From Christoforou J, Balasubramaniam R, Klasser G. Neuropathic orofacial pain. Curr Oral Health Rep 2015;2(3):150; with permission.

ii. Gabapentin, pregabalin, topiramate, or even the older anticonvulsants valproate and phenytoin may be trialed[12]

iii. Botulinum toxin type A[16]

If pharmacologic management fails or there are several side effects that will preclude use, surgical options are instigated (**Table 2**):

1. Microvascular decompression
   a. When there is an identifiable area of vascular compression
2. Gamma knife
   a. When patients are not surgical candidates
3. Other treatments
   a. Balloon compression surgery, nerve sectioning, and ablative options
   b. Low-level laser therapy-insufficient evidence to support its use[32]

Table 2
Surgical options for neuralgia

	TN	GPN	Geniculate Neuralgia	Superior Laryngeal Neuralgia
Microvascular decompression	Immediate pain relief in 88% of patients with 73% pain free with medication after 1 y and stable to 9.7 y[18] Complications: hearing loss[19]	Pain control: 84.7% and recurrence in 7%[20] Complications: transient dysphagia and/or hoarseness (13.2%) and permanent deficits (5.5%)	Limited studies: mainly case studies An excellent outcome was achieved in (71.5%) and 30% retained the result in 12 mo[21] Complications: transient facial paresis	N/A
Rhizotomy/nerve sectioning	80% initial success with 20% failure or recurrence[22] Complications: anesthesia dolorosa, dysesthesia, corneal analgesia, masticatory muscle weakness, keratitis	Pain control in 87.3% and recurrence in 8.2%[19] Complications: glossopharyngeal sensorial deficits Transient dysphagia/hoarseness (25%)[23] Permanent dysphagia, vocal cord paralysis (19.1%)[23]	Limited studies: pain relief was achieved in 72.2%[24] Complications: partial facial paralysis, ipsilateral xerophthalmia	Few studies[25]
Balloon compression	Initial success rate of 85%, but from these patients, it reduces to 36% after 20 mo[26] Complications: visual disturbance, xerophthalmia, anesthesia dolorosa	N/A	N/A	N/A

(continued on next page)

Table 2
(continued)

	TN	GPN	Geniculate Neuralgia	Superior Laryngeal Neuralgia
Ablative options: pulsed radiofrequency neurolysis	High initial pain relief (98%), but 15%–20% show recurrence in 12 mo and 57.7% are pain free after 5 y[27] Complications: diminished corneal reflex, masseter weakness and paralysis, dysesthesia	Pulsed radiofrequency thermocoagulation: 78.8% pain free initially and then 53.2% had an excellent/good pain relief after 5 y[28] Complications: dysesthesia, dysphagia	Uncommon	Uncommon
Stereotactic radiosurgery Cyberknife	Initial success of 75% and 50% are pain free at 3 y[29] 6% facial paraesthesia and 4% hypoesthesia[30]	A failure rate of 40%[31] Minimal reported adverse effects	Uncommon	Uncommon
Stylectomy	N/A	For Eagle syndrome	N/A	N/A

Abbreviation: N/A, not applicable.

Long-term follow-up of patients who have TN shows that well-defined periods of pain attacks are variably followed by periods of remission. However, TN bears a poor prognosis; approximately 90% of patients who have TN report increased attack frequency and severity accompanied by a progressive and increasing resistance to pharmacologic and surgical treatment.[9,33]

GLOSSOPHARYNGEAL NEURALGIA

Glossopharyngeal neuralgia (GPN) is a severe, transient (fraction of a second to 2 minute), stabbing pain experienced in the ear, base of the tongue, tonsillar fossa, or beneath the angle of the jaw.[34] Pain is usually unilateral, but up to 25% of patients may experience bilateral pain.[35]

The overall incidence is estimated to be between 0.2 and 0.7 per 100,000 individuals per year.[35] GPN occurs in adults, with a predilection for women and for patients over the age of 50.[36]

GPN may be divided into the classical and symptomatic types (**Fig. 3**).

Pathogenesis

Most GN patients have no underlying cause or associated neurologic deficit (classical).[34] It is somewhat unclear, but it is thought that the posterior inferior cerebellar artery compresses the glossopharyngeal nerve, with the apex of the loop impinging against the ninth and 10th nerve root entry zones[39] as it exits from the medulla and travels through the subarachnoid space to the jugular foramen.

Clinical Presentation

- Paroxysms of severe, electric shocklike pain in the sensory distribution of the auricular and pharyngeal branches of glossopharyngeal (IX) and vagus (X) cranial nerves.[40]
  - Pain attacks mainly manifest during the day, but can also disturb sleep.
  - Episodes typically last from seconds to minutes.
- Pain is referred to the external ear canal, the base of the ipsilateral tongue, the tonsil, oropharynx, larynx, or the area beneath the angle of the jaw.[36]
- The neuralgic episodes may occur spontaneously, but are usually associated with triggering factors:
  - Chewing, swallowing, coughing, yawning, sneezing, clearing the throat, blowing the nose, rubbing the ear, talking, or laughing.

It may be accompanied by severe cardiovascular issues, such as:

- Life-threatening syncopal episodes
- Hypotension
- Bradycardia
- Asystole

These cardiovascular issues are due to the concomitant involvement of the vagal nerve, which supplies the carotid sinus. Approximately 10% of patients with GPN experience excessive vagal effects during an attack (vagoglossopharyngeal neuralgia).[40]

Diagnosis

The diagnosis of GPN is largely clinical, by the pattern of episodic ear and/or throat pain episodes, triggered by touching the palate or tonsil. There is cessation of pain with topical anesthesia in the area of the pharynx or when the glossopharyngeal nerve is blocked at the jugular foramen.[41]

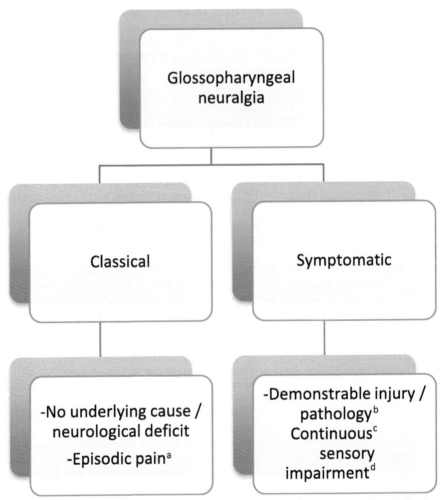

Fig. 3. Classification of GN. [a] A fraction of a second to 2 minutes. [b] Trauma, neoplasm, infection, inflammatory processes,[37] vascular malformation, demyelination, or an elongated styloid process.[38] [c] The aching pain can persist between neuralgic episodes. [d] Numbness can be found in the distribution of the auricular and pharyngeal branches of the vagus nerve as well as branches of the glossopharyngeal nerve.

No imaging findings or other testing has been reliably linked to GPN.[42] Nevertheless, high-resolution MRI or computed tomographic (CT) imaging of the brainstem may reveal the presence of vascular compression, tumors, or demyelinating lesions involving the glossopharyngeal nerve.[23,34,36]

Management

Pharmacologic

Carbamazepine is the first-line agent for GN. Among other anticonvulsants, the most frequently used is phenytoin, lamotrigine, oxcarbazepine, gabapentin, or pregabalin. However, the efficacy of these drugs is variable and could decline over time[40] (see **Table 1**).

When cardiovascular components are associated with the pain, the administration of atropine can be considered to prevent the possible life-threatening cardiac phenomena.[40]

Surgical

Surgical options should be considered in situations of drug intolerance, inefficacy, allergies, or side effects associated with medical therapy.

The treatment of choice for GN caused by a neurovascular conflict (classical) is microvascular decompression. The vessel that most commonly is found to be responsible for the compression is the posterior-inferior cerebellar artery, followed by vertebral artery.[43]

The second-line therapy is a rhizotomy of the IX cranial nerve, although this procedure carries the risk of causing sensorial deficits (see **Table 2**).[23]

Stereotactic radiosurgery, particularly, such as cyberknife, would be indicated for all the patients who are less than ideal candidates for open surgery, due to age or relevant comorbidity.[44]

NERVUS INTERMEDIUS (FACIAL NERVE/GENICULATE NEURALGIA)

Nervus intermedius neuralgia is described as a severe, short-lasting pain in the auditory canal in the absence of other pathologic condition.[34] Nervus intermedius neuralgia is rare. Middle-aged adults seem to be predominantly affected, women more than men.[45]

Clinical Presentation

- Short-lasting (lasting anywhere from seconds to minutes)
- Severe, stabbing pain felt deep in the auditory canal
- Trigger area in the posterior wall of the auditory canal
- Pain can be accompanied by disorders of lacrimation, salivation, and taste[34]

Pathogenesis

The etiology of the pain is largely unknown. Vascular compression by the anterior inferior cerebellar artery, the posterior inferior cerebellar artery, and the branches of the vertebral arteries at the root entry zone of the VIIth and VIIIth cranial nerves may possibly exert pressure on this nerve complex. Nevertheless, in different surgical reports, section or decompression of a combination of cranial nerves V, VII, VIII, IX, X, and/or XI has been necessary to obtain relief.[45]

Diagnosis

A diagnosis of nervus intermedius neuralgia must involve the elimination of all non-neuralgic causes of otalgia (**Fig. 4**).

MRI (of the cerebellopontine angle) with contrast may be used to detect structural pathologic condition, such as a vascular loop compressing the nervus intermedius. There is high sensitivity but poor specificity.[46,47]

Management

Because this condition is relatively uncommon, the literature addressing the efficacy of proposed treatment strategies is scarce.[47]

There are no reports specifically related to the medical therapy for geniculate neuralgia. Pharmacologic treatment is based largely on extrapolation from treatments that are effective for other cranial neuralgias, mainly TN. Hence, a trial of carbamazepine is reasonable for patients with nervus intermedius neuralgia.

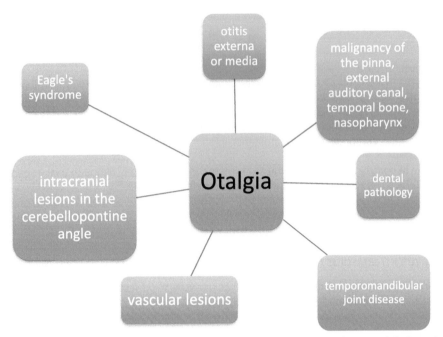

Fig. 4. Nonneuralgic causes of otalgia. (*Adapted from* Tang I, Freeman S, Kontorinis G, et al. Geniculate neuralgia: a systematic review. J Laryngol Otol 2014;128:395; with permission.)

Surgical options are effective in patients for whom medical therapy has failed; nevertheless, management is based on case reports and small series.[48]

Most studies in the literature support microvascular decompression at its root entry zone to the brainstem if compression by a vascular loop is present, or nerve section, intracranially. Nevertheless, well-designed prospective studies looking at the efficacy of microsurgery and nerve sectioning in terms of pain relief and quality of life are needed.[48]

SUPERIOR LARYNGEAL NEURALGIA

Superior laryngeal neuralgia is a rare disorder, with short-lasting pain, localized predominantly to one side of the laryngeal region and occasionally radiating to the lower lateral jaw or ear[49]:

- Paroxysmal pain
- Lancinating pain
- May be triggered by pressure to the skin above and lateral to the thyroid cartilage where the internal branch of the superior laryngeal nerve pierces the thyrohyoid membrane

Pathogenesis

The causes of superior laryngeal neuralgia can be classified as either central or peripheral (**Fig. 5**).

The etiology is unclear, but may be associated with the following:

- Deviation of the hyoid bone
- Lateral pharyngeal diverticulum[50]

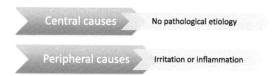

Fig. 5. Causes of superior laryngeal neuralgia.

- Trauma
- A minor upper respiratory tract disease or a viral infection, such as influenza, laryngitis[51]
- Previous tonsillectomy[49]
- Compression of the nerve by the superior thyroid artery and/or vein

Clinical Presentation

- Sharp, searing pain
- Pain lasts for minutes to hours
- Pain may radiate to the posterior auricular area
- A trigger point often within the larynx (lateral aspect of the throat overlying the thyrohyoid membrane)
  - Swallowing
    - May lead to the patient avoiding food and result in significant weight loss
  - Straining the voice, singing
  - Turning of the head

Diagnosis

Patients must respond to a local superior laryngeal nerve anesthetic block to be diagnosed with superior laryngeal neuralgia according to the criteria of the second edition of the *International Classification of Headache Disorders*.[52] Anesthetizing the larynx with topical anesthetic is an alternative method for confirming the diagnosis.[53]

CT scanning of the larynx can be performed to rule out any pathologic conditions in laryngeal and perilaryngeal structures.[54]

Management

1. Carbamazepine is the most commonly used medication with good effectiveness reported, although failures have been reported.[55]
2. Regional blockage of laryngeal nerve: Repeated injections of local anesthetics have been noted to be an effective treatment in isolated cases.[56]
3. Nerve section has been uniformly effective.

PERIPHERAL NEURITIS

Neuritis is a localized neural pathologic condition resulting from inflammation.

Pathogenesis

- It may arise from direct axonal damage
  - Misdirected dental implant, periapical dental inflammatory lesion near a nerve
- A result of cytokine secretion
  - A temporomandibular joint pathologic condition,[57] paranasal sinusitis,[58] malignancies[59]

Persistence of the perineural inflammation along a nerve is as a result of macrophage and lymphocyte recruitment. There is an increase in tumor necrosis factor-α, which increases Na^+ conductance in cell membranes, hence resulting in spontaneous nociceptor activity at axons.[60]

Clinical Presentation

- Tactile allodynia
  - May occur a few hours following nerve exposure to the inflammatory process[60] and may last for several days[60]
  - Hypersensitivity usually peaks at 1 week and may decrease at 1 month.[60] Nevertheless, the neural inflammation plays a role in triggering and maintaining neuropathic pain and hence, in some individuals, symptoms can continue for years[60]

Diagnosis

Diagnosis is largely based on clinical history, clinical examination, and investigations, such as radiological imaging and pathologic workup (B12 deficiency, viral infection, autoimmunity) to identify the inflammatory contributor.

Management

Management aims to decrease perineural and neural inflammation. Early administration of corticosteroids or nonsteroidal anti-inflammatory drugs (NSAIDs) may offer benefit.

HERPES ZOSTER AND POSTHERPETIC NEURALGIA

Herpes zoster (HZ) results from the reactivation of the varicella zoster virus (VZV) within the cranial sensory ganglia. This viral reactivation leads to acute inflammatory changes within the ganglion of the affected dermatome but also extends peripherally along the length of the sensory nerve (neuritis), followed by neuronal destruction.[61] These inflammatory changes and neural damage results in a painful vesicular rash in the associated unilateral dermatome.

HZ has a prodrome of less than a week. The pain may be described as throbbing and burning, which intensifies with stress and tiredness.

HZ presents more commonly in patients affected by autoimmune disease,[62] or immune suppressed states such as in patients with cancer, transplant patients, the elderly, and those experiencing excessive stress.[63]

Antiviral therapy may reduce symptoms when used within 72 hours of rash onset (Box 1). Other medications that may aid in pain management include tricyclic antidepressants, gabapentinoids, and opioids.[64]

Vaccinating individuals who are at risk, such as those who are elderly and immunocompromised, may be an efficacious technique to prevent HZ and PHN.[65]

Postherpetic Neuralgia

A proportion (16%–22%) of patients who have acute HZ will report pain 3 to 6 months after initial onset, and these are categorized as having PHN. Trigeminal PHN is a direct complication of acute HZ of the trigeminal nerve and will therefore localize to the affected dermatome.

Box 1
Antiviral recommendation

- Valacyclovir (1000 mg 3 times a day for 7 days)
- Acyclovir (800 mg 5 times a day for 7 days)
- Famciclovir (500 mg 3 times a day for 7 days)

Clinical

- Pain in PHN is burning, throbbing, stabbing, shooting, or sharp.
- Itching of affected areas is common in trigeminal dermatomes and may be prominent and bothersome.
- PHN is usually severe.
- The symptoms are characterized by fluctuations.

Pathogenesis

PHN is a neuropathic pain syndrome resulting from viral-induced nerve injury. Scarring of sensory ganglia, peripheral nerves, and loss of large myelinated fibers is commonly found in patients who have PHN.[66]

PHN is thought to progress from peripheral to central structures. Ongoing activity in peripheral nociceptors has been shown to be important in the early stages (<1 year) of PHN, whereas central mechanisms may become prominent in later stages.[67]

Management

The first-line treatment options include amitriptyline and nortriptyline and gabapentin or pregabalin (**Table 3**).

These can also be combined with the following:
- Opioids (oxycodone, morphine, or tramadol)
- Topical transdermal therapies

Low-level laser therapy is seen in the literature, but there is insufficient evidence to support its use.[78]

Unfortunately, in the older age group (>60 years), 50% or more will continue to experience pain lasting more than 1 year.[79] Management is challenging with much of the treatment not being completely effective.

PERSISTENT IDIOPATHIC FACIAL PAIN

Persistent idiopathic facial pain (PIFP) refers to persistent extraoral and/or intraoral pain along the territory of the trigeminal nerve that does not fit the classic presentation of other cranial neuralgias or another disorder.[80] PIFP is mainly seen in adult women with a prevalence of 0.03 to 1.0%.[80]

Clinical

- Pain is of long duration (if not continuous)
- Unilateral
- Severe ache, crushing, or burning sensation
- No sensory loss
- Poorly localized
- Patients may complain of other symptoms
  - Headache, backache, irritable bowel, uterine bleeding

Diagnosis

Other facial pains must be excluded when making a diagnosis. For example, conditions such as temporal arteritis may need to be excluded in patients older than 50 years by appropriate investigations.

In addition, Forssell and colleagues,[81] when comparing patients with trigeminal neuropathic pain with PIFP, showed that up to 75% of patients with PIFP

Table 3
Medications for continuous neuropathic pain

	Medication	Other Remarks
PIFP	1. Amitriptyline (25–100 mg/d)[68] 2. Serotonin–norepinephrine reuptake inhibitors (venlafaxine[69] and duloxetine[70]) These can be used in combination with: • Gabapentin (900–1800 mg/d) • Pregabalin (150–300 mg/d) Topical formulations, such as lidocaine transdermal (5%) anesthetic, may also be trialed[71]	A multidisciplinary approach encompassing the comorbidities is suggested: • Mindfulness • Meditation • Yoga • Sleep hygiene • Cognitive behavioral therapy
Peripheral painful traumatic trigeminal neuropathy	Tricyclic antidepressants (TCA) or gabapentinoids are first line (TCAs have had increased study but there are reduced side effects with pregabalin and gabapentin) Further benefits may be attained with opioids or tramadol or newer agents such as duloxetine[72] Topical medication as single treatment or in combination with systemic medications can be trialed[73] If episodic (rather than chronic): a combination of a corticosteroid (prednisone 60 mg daily) with pregabalin (150 mg twice daily) was found to be effective[74]	
Postherpetic neuralgia	• Amitriptyline (start 10 – 25 mg nightly then up to 75 – 150mg/d maintenance)[75] or • Nortriptyline (start 10 – 25 mg nightly then up to 75 – 150mg/d maintenance)[75] or • Gabapentin (start 100 mg 3 times a day then up to 1800mg/d maintenance)[75] or Pregabalin (start 50 – 75 mg 2 times a day then up to 600mg/d maintenance)[75] If lack of response: • Opioids (oxycodone, morphine, 5–15 mg 4 hourly as needed),[75] or • Tramadol (50 mg every 4–6 h)[75] Topical (transdermal) therapies: lidocaine 5%[76] or 8% capsaicin patches[77]	Early management of HZ improves prognosis of PHN
Peripheral neuritis	Corticosteroids NSAIDs	

demonstrated abnormalities on neurophysiologic testing. Hence, it is important that these patients have some form of psychological testing.[82]

Pathogenesis

The pathophysiology is largely unknown; nevertheless, PIFP appears to be multifactorial with traumatic, psychological, and neurobiological influences. Patients with PIFP have brain morphology changes consistent with those who have chronic pain,[83] but studies suggest that somatosensory processing is not used to maintain the pain.[84]

Management

Management revolves around improving a patient's quality of life by balancing pain control with medication side effects. Hence, a multidisciplinary approach is usually undertaken.

Some selective serotonin reuptake inhibitors or selective noradrenalin and serotonin inhibitors are used and usually long term.[85] Anticonvulsant drugs have not been shown to be effective.

Improved sleep hygiene, which can reduce pain vulnerability, and techniques, such as mindfulness, meditation, and yoga, can be helpful. Hence, techniques such as cognitive behavior therapy are likely to have a positive outcome.[86]

Harrison and colleagues[87] showed that the best outcomes were obtained with a combination of an antidepressant with cognitive behavior therapy.

Low-level laser therapy has been trialed, but there is insufficient evidence to support its use.[88]

PERIPHERAL PAINFUL TRAUMATIC TRIGEMINAL NEUROPATHY

Peripheral painful traumatic trigeminal neuropathy is defined as a spontaneous or stimulus-dependent pain or disturbed sensation, predominately affecting the receptive field of one or more divisions of the trigeminal nerve.

There is a combination of environmental (reduced social support),[89] psychosocial (anxious, introverted personalities),[89] and genetic factors (polymorphism in the gene encoding serotonin transporter),[72,89] which may vary an individual's pain experience.

Clinical

- Signs of trigeminal nerve dysfunction
  - Positive (hyperalgesia, allodynia) and/or
  - Negative (hypoesthesia, hypoalgesia)
- Typically moderate to severe pain
  - Burning, stabbing[72]
- Most cases are continuous but may be episodic (minutes to days).
- The pain distribution may spread with time due to central mechanisms but usually remains unilateral

Diagnosis

A thorough history, clinical examination, and adjunctive investigations are required to exclude pathologic condition, such as nerve impingement, infections, and neoplastic lesions.

Pathogenesis

The neuropathy typically develops within 3 months of an identifiable, traumatic event to the painful region. The neuropathy may be due to the following[72]:

- Minor oral interventions
  - Extractions, endodontic treatment, and implant placement
- Major craniofacial injury

Following injury to the trigeminal branches, chronic pain develops in about 3% to 5% of patients.[90] The tissue injury results in the release of inflammatory mediators and nerve damage with the establishment of peripheral sensitization.[91] Repeated nociceptive sensory input leads to the establishment of central sensitization.[72]

Management

Pharmacologic management is with the use of tricyclic antidepressants, serotonin norepinephrine reuptake inhibitors, or gabapentinoids.[92] Opioids may also be incorporated in these regimes (see **Table 3**).[72]

The efficacy of surgery remains unclear due to insufficient trials.[72]

SUMMARY

Further research is required to further the knowledge of neuropathic orofacial pain conditions as well as their management.

Newer therapies are currently being tested, such as novel cellular/molecular therapies, for neuropathic orofacial pain disorders, including local injection of autologous mesenchymal stem cells,[93] regulation of satellite glial cells,[94] and delivery of substance P,[95] endomorphin,[96] and cannabinoids.[97]

Well-constructed trials are required to introduce more effective management options for neuropathic orofacial pain patients.

REFERENCES

1. Fromm GH, Graff-Radford SB, Terrence CF, et al. Pre-trigeminal neuralgia. Neurology 1990;40:1493–5.
2. Puca A, Meglio M, Vari R, et al. Evaluation of fifth nerve dysfunction in 136 patients with middle and posterior cranial fossae tumors. Eur Neurol 1995;35:33–7.
3. De Simone R, Marano E, Brescia Morra V, et al. A clinical comparison of trigeminal neuralgic pain in patients with and without underlying multiple sclerosis. Neurol Sci 2005;26:s150–1.
4. Tyler-Kabara EC, Kassam AB, Horowitz MH, et al. Predictors of outcome in surgically managed patients with typical and atypical trigeminal neuralgia: comparison of results following microvascular decompression. J Neurosurg 2002;96:527–31.
5. Sato J, Saitoh T, Notani K, et al. Diagnostic significance of carbamazepine and trigger zones in trigeminal neuralgia. Oral Surg Oral Med Oral Pathol Oral Radiol Endod 2004;97:18–22.
6. Devor M, Amir R. Pathophysiology of trigeminal neuralgia: the ignition hypothesis. Clin J Pain 2002;18:4–13.
7. Benoliel R, Eliav E. Neuropathic orofacial pain. Oral Maxillofac Surg Clin North Am 2008;20(2):237–54.
8. Jorns T, Zakrzewska J. Evidence based approach to the medical management of trigeminal neuralgia. Br J Neurosurg 2007;21:253–61.
9. Zakrzewska J, Patsalos P. Long-term cohort study comparing medical (oxcarbazepine) and surgical management of intractable trigeminal neuralgia. Pain 2002;95:259–66.
10. Zakrzewska J, Chaudhry Z, Nurmikko T, et al. Lamotrigine (lamictal) in refractory trigeminal neuralgia: results from a double-blind placebo controlled crossover trial. Pain 1997;73:223–30.
11. Fromm G, Terrence C, Chattha A. Baclofen in the treatment of trigeminal neuralgia: double-blind study and long-term follow-up. Ann Neurol 1984;15:240–4.
12. Cheshire WP. Defining the role for gabapentin in the treatment of trigeminal neuralgia: a retrospective study. J Pain 2002;3:137–42.
13. Obermann M, Yoon MS, Sensen K, et al. Efficacy of pregabalin in the treatment of trigeminal neuralgia. Cephalalgia 2008;28:174–81.

14. Zvartau-Hind M, Din M, Gilani A, et al. Topiramate relieves refractory trigeminal neuralgia in MS patients. Neurology 2000;55:1587–8.
15. Kanai A, Saito M, Hoka S. Subcutaneous sumatriptan for refractory trigeminal neuralgia. Headache 2006;46:577–82.
16. Morra M, Elgebaly A, Elmaraezy A, et al. Therapeutic efficacy and safety of botulinum toxin A therapy in trigeminal neuralgia: a systematic review and meta-analysis of randomized controlled trials. J Headache Pain 2016;17:63.
17. Verma G. Role of botulinum toxin type-A (BTX-A) in the management of trigeminal neuralgia. Pain Res Treat 2013;2013:831094.
18. Oesman C, Mooij J. Long-term follow-up of microvascular decompression for trigeminal neuralgia. Skull Base 2011;21:313–22.
19. Sarsam Z, Garcia-Fiana M, Nurmikko TJ, et al. The long-term outcome of microvascular decompression for trigeminal neuralgia. Br J Neurosurg 2010;24(1):18–25.
20. Rey-Dios R, Cohen-Gadol AA. Current neurosurgical management of glossopharyngeal neuralgia and technical nuances for microvascular decompression surgery. Neurosurg Focus 2013;34:E8.
21. Lovely TJ, Jannetta PJ. Surgical management of geniculate neuralgia. Am J Otol 1997;18(4):512–7.
22. Nanjappa M, Kumaraswamy SV, Keerthi R, et al. Percutaneous radiofrequency rhizotomy in treatment of trigeminal neuralgia: a prospective study. J Maxillofac Oral Surg 2013;12(1):35–41.
23. Alafaci C, Granata F, Cutugno M, et al. Glossopharyngeal neuralgia caused by a complex neurovascular conflict: case report and review of the literature. Surg Neurol Int 2015;6:19.
24. Rupa V, Saunders RL, Weider DJ. Geniculate neuralgia: the surgical management of primary otalgia. J Neurosurg 1991;75:505–11.
25. Zong Q, Zhang K, Han G, et al. Rhizotomy targeting the intermediate nerve, the glossopharyngeal nerve and the upper 1st to 2nd rootlets of the vagus nerve for the treatment of laryngeal neuralgia combined with intermediate nerve neuralgia-a case report. BMC Surg 2014;14:60.
26. Kouzounias K, Schechtmann G, Lind G, et al. Factors that influence outcome of percutaneous balloon compression in the treatment of trigeminal neuralgia. Neurosurgery 2010;67:925–34.
27. Kanpolat Y, Savas A, Bekar A, et al. Percutaneous controlled radiofrequency trigeminal rhizotomy for the treatment of idiopathic trigeminal neuralgia: 25-year experience with 1,600 patients. Neurosurgery 2001;48:524–32.
28. Wang X, Tang Y, Zeng Y, et al. Long-term outcomes of percutaneous radiofrequency thermocoagulation for glossopharyngeal neuralgia A retrospective observational study. Medicine (Baltimore) 2016;95(48):e5530.
29. Lopez B, Hamlyn P, Zakrzewska J. Stereotactic radiosurgery for primary trigeminal neuralgia: state of the evidence and recommendation for future reports. J Neurol Neurosurg Psychiatry 2004;75:1019–24.
30. Régis J, Metellus P, Hayashi M, et al. Prospective controlled trial of gamma knife surgery for essential trigeminal neuralgia. J Neurosurg 2006;104(6):913–24.
31. Pollock BE, Boes C. Stereotactic Radiosurgery for Glossopharyngeal Neuralgia: preliminary report of 5 cases. J Neurosurg 2011;115:936–9.
32. Falaki F, Nejat AH, Dalirsani Z. The effect of low-level laser therapy on trigeminal neuralgia: a review of literature. J Dent Res Dent Clin Dent Prospects 2014;8(1):1–5.
33. Bowsher D. Trigeminal neuralgia: a symptomatic study of 126 successive patients with and without previous interventions. Pain Clinic 2000;12:93–101.

34. Headache Classification Subcommittee of the International Headache Society. The international classification of headache disorders, 3rd edition (beta version). Cephalalgia 2013;33(9):629–808.
35. Katusic S, Williams DB, Beard CM, et al. Incidence and clinical features of glossopharyngeal neuralgia, Rochester, Minnesota, 1945-1984. Neuroepidemiology 1991;10(5–6):266–75.
36. Rozen TD. Trigeminal neuralgia and glossopharyngeal neuralgia. Neurol Clin 2004;22(1):185–206.
37. Urban PP, Keilmann A, Teichmann EM. Sensory neuropathy of the trigeminal, glossopharyngeal, and vagal nerves in Sjögren's syndrome. J Neurol Sci 2001; 186(1–2):59–63.
38. Singh PM, Kaur M, Trikha A. An uncommonly common: glossopharyngeal neuralgia. Ann Indian Acad Neurol 2013;16(1):1–8.
39. Zhao H, Zhang X, Zhu J, et al. Microvascular decompression for glossopharyngeal neuralgia: long-term follow-up. World Neurosurg 2017;102:151–6.
40. Blumenfeld A, Nikolskaya G. Glossopharyngeal neuralgia. Curr Pain Headache Rep 2013;17:343.
41. de Leon-Casasola O. New developments in the treatment algorithm for peripheral neuropathic pain. Pain Med 2011;12(supp3):s100–8.
42. Burchiel KJ. Glossopharyngeal neuralgia. J Neurosurg 2011;115(5):934–5.
43. Franzini A, Messina G, Franzini A, et al. Treatments of glossopharyngeal neuralgia: towards standard procedures. Neurol Sci 2017;38(supp1):51–5.
44. Franzini A, Ferroli P, Messina G, et al. Surgical treatment of cranial neuralgias. Handb Clin Neurol 2010;97:679–92.
45. Bruyn G. Nervus intermedius neuralgia (Hunt). Cephalalgia 1984;4:71.
46. Tang I, Freeman S, Kontorinis G, et al. Geniculate neuralgia: a systematic review. J Laryngol Otol 2014;128:394–9.
47. Saers S, Han K, de Ru J. Microvascular decompression may be an effective treatment for nervus intermedius neuralgia. J Laryngol Otol 2011;125:520–2.
48. Tubbs R, Steck D, Mortazavi M, et al. The nervus intermedius: a review of its anatomy, function, pathology, and role in neurosurgery. World Neurosurg 2013; 79(5–6):763–7.
49. Bruyn GW. Superior laryngeal neuralgia. Cephalalgia 1983;3:235–40.
50. Bagatzounis A. Lateral pharyngeal diverticulum as a cause of superior laryngeal nerve neuralgia. Laryngorhinootologie 1994;73(4):219–21.
51. Amin MR, Koufman JA. Vagal neuropathy after upper respiratory infection: a viral etiology? Am J Otolaryngol 2001;22(4):251–6.
52. Headache Classification Subcommittee of the International Headache Society. The international classification of headache disorders: 2nd edition. Cephalalgia 2004;24(supp1):9–160.
53. Kodama S, Oribe K, Suzuki M. Superior laryngeal neuralgia associated with deviation of the hyoid bone. Auris Nasus Larynx 2008;35:429–31.
54. Aydin O, Ozturk M, Anik Y. Superior laryngeal neuralgia after acute laryngitis and treatment with a single injection of a local anesthetic. Arch Otolaryngol Head Neck Surg 2007;133:934–5.
55. Brownstone PK, Ballenger JJ, Vick NA. Bilateral superior laryngeal neuralgia: its successful treatment with carbamazepine. Arch Neurol 1980;37:525.
56. Takahashi SK, Suzuki M, Izuha A, et al. Two cases of idiopathic superior laryngeal neuralgia treated by superior laryngeal nerve block with a high concentration of lidocaine. J Clin Anesth 2007;19:237–8.

57. Eliav E, Teich S, Nitzan D, et al. Facial arthralgia and myalgia: can they be differentiated by trigeminal sensory assessment? Pain 2003;104:481–90.

58. Benoliel R, Biron A, Quek SY, et al. Trigeminal neurosensory changes following acute and chronic paranasal sinusitis. Quintessence Int 2006;37(6):437–43.

59. Eliav E, Teich S, Benoliel R, et al. Large myelinated nerve fiber hypersensitivity in oral malignancy. Oral Surg Oral Med Oral Pathol Oral Radiol Endod 2002;94: 45–50.

60. Bove G, Ransil B, Lin H, et al. Inflammation induces ectopic mechanical sensitivity in axons of nociceptors innervating deep tissues. J Neurophysiol 2003;90: 1949–55.

61. Wood M. Understanding pain in herpes zoster: an essential for optimizing treatment. J Infect Dis 2002;186:S78–82.

62. Rondaan C, de Haan A, Horst G, et al. Altered cellular and humoral immunity to varicella-zoster virus in patients with autoimmune diseases. Arthritis Rheumatol 2014;66:3122–8.

63. Coughlin S. Anxiety and depression: linkages with viral diseases. Public Health Rev 2012;34:1–15.

64. Dworkin R, Johnson R, Breuer J, et al. Recommendations for the management of herpes zoster. Clin Infect Dis 2007;44:S1–26.

65. Oxman MN, Levin MJ, Johnson GR, et al. A vaccine to prevent herpes zoster and postherpetic neuralgia in older adults. N Engl J Med 2005;352:2271–84.

66. Watson CP, Deck JH, Morshead C, et al. Post-herpetic neuralgia: further postmortem studies of cases with and without pain. Pain 1991;44:105–17.

67. Pappagallo M, Oaklander AL, Quatrano-Piacentini AL, et al. Heterogenous patterns of sensory dysfunction in postherpetic neuralgia suggest multiple pathophysiologic mechanisms. Anesthesiology 2000;92:691–8.

68. Pettengill CA, Reisner-Keller L. The use of tricyclic antidepressants for the control of chronic orofacial pain. Cranio 1997;15:53–6.

69. Forssell H, Tasmuth T, Tenovuo O, et al. Venlafaxine in the treatment of atypical facial pain: a randomized controlled trial. J Orofac Pain 2004;18:131–7.

70. Nagashima W, Kimura H, Ito M, et al. Effectiveness of duloxetine for the treatment of chronic nonorganic orofacial pain. Clin Neuropharmacol 2012;35:273–7.

71. Cornelissen P, van Kleef M, Mekhail N, et al. Evidence-based interventional pain medicine according to clinical diagnoses 3. Persistent idiopathic facial pain. Pain Pract 2009;9:443–8.

72. Benoliel R, Kahn J, Eliav E. Peripheral painful traumatic trigeminal neuropathies. Oral Dis 2012;18:317–32.

73. Heir G, Karolchek S, Kalladka M, et al. Use of topical medication in orofacial neuropathic pain: a retrospective study. Oral Surg Oral Med Oral Pathol Oral Radiol Endod 2008;105:466–9.

74. Lopez-Lopez J, Estrugo-Devesa A, Jane-Salas E, et al. Medical treatment of post-dental extraction peripheral painful traumatic trigeminal neuropathy. Quintessence Int 2013;44:703–6.

75. Johnson RW, Rice ASC. Clinical practice. Postherpetic neuralgia. N Engl J Med 2014;371:1526–33.

76. Dworkin R, Backonja M, Rowbotham M, et al. Advances in neuropathic pain: diagnosis mechanisms and treatment recommendations. Arch Neurol 2003;60: 1524–34.

77. Wallace MS, Pappagallo M. Qutenza: a capsaicin 8% patch for the management of postherpetic neuralgia. Expert Rev Neurother 2011;11:15–27.

78. Knapp DJ. Postherpetic neuralgia: case study of class 4 laser therapy intervention. Clin J Pain 2013;29(10):e6–9.
79. Philip A, Thakur R. Postherpetic neuralgia. J Palliat Med 2011;14:765–73.
80. Klasser G. Management of persistent idiopathic orofacial pain. J Can Dent Assoc 2013;79:d71.
81. Forssell H, Tenovuo O, Silvoniemi P, et al. Differences and similarities between atypical facial pain and trigeminal neuropathic pain. Neurology 2007;69:1451–9.
82. Zakrzewska J. Chronic/persistent idiopathic facial pain. Neurosurg Clin N Am 2016;27(3):345–51.
83. Schmidt-Wilcke T, Hierlmeier S, Leinisch E. Altered regional brain morphology in patients with chronic facial pain. Headache 2010;50:1278–85.
84. Lang E, Kaltenhauser M, Seidler S, et al. Persistent idiopathic facial pain exists independent of somatosensory input from the painful region: findings from quantitative sensory functions and somatotopy of the primary somatosensory cortex. Pain 2005;118:80–91.
85. Feinmann C. The long-term outcome of facial pain treatment. J Psychosom Res 1993;37:381–7.
86. Morley S, Eccleston C, Williams A. Systematic review and meta-analysis of randomized controlled trials of cognitive behaviour therapy and behaviour therapy for chronic pain in adults, excluding headache. Pain 1999;80:1–13.
87. Harrison SD, Glover L, Feinmann C, et al. A comparison of antidepressant medication alone and in conjunction with cognitive behavioural therapy for chronic idiopathic facial pain. In: Jensen TS, Turner JA, Wiesenfeld Z, editors. Proceedings of the 8th World Congress on pain, progress in pain research and management. Seattle (WA): IASP Press; 1997. p. 663–72.
88. Yang HW, Huang YF. Treatment of persistent idiopathic facial pain (PIFP) with a low-level energy diode laser. Photomed Laser Surg 2011;29(10):701–10.
89. Edwards R. Individual differences in endogenous pain modulation as a risk factor for chronic pain. Neurology 2005;65:437–43.
90. Jaaskelainen SK, Teerijoki-Oksa T, Virtanen A, et al. Sensory regeneration following intraoperatively verified trigeminal nerve injury. Neurology 2004;62: 1951–7.
91. Neumann S, Doubell T, Leslie T, et al. Inflammatory pain hypersensitivity mediated by phenotypic switch in myelinated primary sensory neuron. Nature 1996; 384:360–4.
92. Finnerup N, Sindrup S. The evidence of pharmacological treatment of neuropathic pain. Pain 2010;150:573–81.
93. Vickers ER, Karsten E, Flood J, et al. A preliminary report on stem cell therapy for neuropathic pain in humans. J Pain Res 2014;7:255–63.
94. Ohara PT, Vit J, Bhargava A, et al. Gliopathic pain: when satellite glial cells go bad. Neuroscientist 2009;15(5):450–63.
95. Mustafa G, Anderson EM, Bokrand-Donatelli Y, et al. Anti-nociceptive effect of a conjugate of substance P and light chain of botulinum neurotoxin type A. Pain 2013;154(11):2547–53.
96. Makuch W, Mika J, Rojewska E, et al. Effects of selective and non-selective inhibitors of nitric oxide synthase on morphine- and endomorphin-1-induced analgesia in acute and neuropathic pain in rats. Neuropharmacology 2013;75:445–57.
97. Rahn EJ, Hohmann AG. Cannabinoids as pharmacotherapies for neuropathic pain: From the bench to the bedside. Neurotherapeutics 2009;6(4):713–37.

Burning Mouth Syndrome

Steven D. Bender, DDS

KEYWORDS

- Burning mouth syndrome • Glossodynia • Oral burning • Neuropathic • Neuropathy

KEY POINTS

- Burning mouth syndrome (BMS) is an idiopathic, poorly understood pain disorder characterized by a burning sensation of the oral cavity in the absence of any identifiable organic disease.
- BMS is most prevalent in postmenopausal women.
- The presentation of BMS can vary from patient to patient, creating a diagnostic challenge for the practitioner.
- Therapies for BMS to date target symptom relief as opposed to providing a cure.
- Translational research of BMS is desperately needed.

INTRODUCTION

Burning mouth syndrome (BMS) is a poorly understood, idiopathic chronic pain disorder that can be characterized by a burning sensation of the oral cavity in the absence of any identifiable organic disease. This syndrome seems more prevalent in menopausal women, with some studies showing comorbid psychosocial and psychiatric disorders.[1,2] The pain presentation is mostly continuous and ranges from moderate to severe in intensity. The American Academy of Orofacial Pain[3] defines BMS as a burning sensation in the oral mucosa despite the absence of clinical findings and abnormalities in laboratory testing or imaging. The International Association for the Study of Pain[4] defines BMS as a burning pain in the tongue or other oral mucous membrane associated with normal signs and laboratory findings lasting at least 4 months to 6 months. In a section described as "painful cranial neuropathies, other facial pains," the *International Headache Society in the International Classification of Headache Disorders*, 3rd edition (beta version) (ICHD-3 beta)[5] defines BMS as an intraoral burning or dysesthetic sensation, recurring daily for more than 2 hours per day over more than 3 months, without clinically evident causative lesions. It becomes apparent that most accepted definitions of this syndrome include reference to a lack of clinical findings that may provide an etiologic explanation. The use of the term, *syndrome*, refers

Disclosure Statement: The author has nothing to disclose.
Facial Pain and Sleep Medicine, Department of Oral and Maxillofacial Surgery, Texas A&M College of Dentistry, 3302 Gaston Avenue, Dallas, TX 75246, USA
E-mail address: bender@tamhsc.edu

Dent Clin N Am 62 (2018) 585–596
https://doi.org/10.1016/j.cden.2018.05.006
0011-8532/18/© 2018 Elsevier Inc. All rights reserved.

to features, such as dryness of the mouth, alteration of salivary function, and taste disturbances, which commonly accompany the burning sensation.[1] Other terminology previously used to describe BMS includes glossodynia, glossalgia, stomatodynia, and sore or burning tongue, among many others.[6,7] Several classification systems have been proposed based on pattern and intensity,[8,9] whether primary or secondary[7] and pathophysiologic mechanisms[10] but, to date, none has been validated.

EPIDEMIOLOGY

The prevalence of BMS reported for the general population varies between 0.7% and 15% and seems to depend on the diagnostic criteria used.[1,11] BMS seems most prevalent in postmenopausal women, although younger women as well as men can also be affected.[1] Most reports suggest a female-to-male ratio of 1:5 to 1:7.[11,12] Prevalence does seem to increase with age in both male and female subjects.[13]

CLINICAL PRESENTATIONS

The clinical presentations of BMS are typically not consistent and vary from patient to patient. The onset of pain may be gradual or sudden, typically with no identifiable precipitating factors. In some cases, however, it can be traced to a precipitating event, such as a dental procedure, trauma, introduction of a new medication, illness, or stressful life event. At presentation, patients usually complain of chronic pain of 4 months to 6 months duration and describe it as annoying, burning or scalding, tingling, or sometimes itchy or numb.[14] Most patients report they experience mild to moderate levels of pain that may be present at awakening or, as in most cases, develops and intensifies as the day progresses.[15,16] Patients often report eating, drinking, and talking can affect their symptoms. In some cases, eating temporarily decreases or aborts the symptoms.[17,18] Most patients, however, avoid hot, spicy, or acidic food/liquids or alcoholic beverages, because they tend to intensify their symptoms. Some patients also report the pain increases or seems more noticeable when they feel more stressed or fatigued. The pain can be continuous or intermittent and is typically localized to the tongue (67.9%), usually the anterior two-thirds, but may involve other mucosal surfaces, such as the palate, lip, buccal mucosa, and floor of the mouth.[19] The pain tends to present bilaterally and symmetrically more so than unilaterally.[20] Occasionally, other body sites are affected, such as the anogenital region. BMS associated with vulvodynia has been reported in the literature.[20,21]

ASSOCIATED FEATURES

In addition to the burning sensation, many patients also complain of dry mouth (xerostomia) and taste alterations. It has been reported that more than two-thirds of BMS patients report dry mouth at presentation.[22] Two recent studies did show a marked reduction in basal salivary flow in subjects with BMS compared with healthy subjects.[23,24] Alterations of taste as well as phantom tastes and smells have been reported by 11% to 69% of BMS patients.[16,19,25] Alterations, such as sour and bitter taste perceived as stronger, sweet tastes perceived as weaker, and salty tastes perceived as weaker or stronger are commonly reported.[16]

Psychosocial and psychological comorbidities have been reported to occur in 85% of BMS patients.[26,27] Anxiety and/or depression, somatization, hypochondria, cancer phobia, and insomnia are the most common diagnoses seen in this patient population. Carlson and colleagues,[28] however, using the Multidimensional Pain Inventory (MPI) and Symptom Checklist–90–Revised (SCL-90R) on 33 BMS cases, concluded that

BMS patients reported significantly fewer disruptions in normal activities as a result of their oral burning pain than did a large sample of other chronic pain patients.

ETIOLOGY

Although the etiology remains mostly unknown, the ICHD-3 beta suggests BMS is a neuropathy.[5] It is commonly accepted that the etiology of BMS is multifactorial and involves the interaction between local and systemic entities.

Local Factors

Local factors, such as odontogenic or mucosal disease; mechanical or chemical irritation; hypersensitivity reactions; viral, fungal, or bacterial infection; and xerostomia, can produce oral burning by direct irritation of the tongue and other oral mucosal surfaces.[11,29,30]

Systemic Factors

Several systemic factors have been suggested as least partially responsible for BMS. Evidence to support these factors, however, is not conclusive in the literature. Systemic factors to be considered include nutritional and vitamin deficiencies, such as vitamin B_{12}, folic acid, iron, and zinc.[31,32] Autoimmune, gastrointestinal, and endocrine disorders, such as diabetes and thyroid dysfunction, have been suggested as well.[33,34] Pharmacotherapeutic agents like angiotensin-converting enzyme inhibitors, including captopril, enalapril, and lisinopril, also deserve consideration.[35,36]

PATHOPHYSIOLOGY

The pathophysiology of BMS has remained mostly unknown over time. It is probable and most likely that it manifests as a result of multiple factors, including the interaction of psychological entities with neurophysiologic factors.

Taste and Sensory System Interactions

It has been suggested that 1 cause of BMS may be the loss of inhibition on the trigeminal nerve as a result of damage to the chorda tympani nerve.[37] Bartoshuk and colleagues[38] previously demonstrated the convergence of taste sensation with pain in both clinical and experimental settings. The chorda tympani nerve, a branch of the facial nerve, supplies taste sensation to the anterior two-thirds of the tongue. It has been shown that unilateral damage to the chorda tympani nerve can result in an increased burning sensation in response to capsaicin applied on the contralateral side to the damage.[39] Bartoshuk and colleagues[37] also demonstrated that individuals who have the genetically determined ability to taste 6-n-propylthiouracil, known as supertasters, tend to a have lowered acceptance of some bitter foods and perceive more burn from irritants, such as capsaicin.[40] Their work suggests this phenomenon is directly related to the density of taste receptors on the anterior tongue. This phenomenon was shown more prevalent in women. In addition, other studies have demonstrated that those with a higher density of taste buds tend to be more prone to developing BMS.[37,41]

Hormonal Alterations

Menopause

Because BMS primarily effects postmenopausal women, some investigators have suggested that altered levels of female sex hormones in the perimenopause to postmenopausal period may predispose women to develop BMS.[7,42] Gao and colleagues[42] found a significantly higher level of follicular stimulating hormone and a lower level of estradiol in blood analyses of patients with BMS compared with controls. Because both BMS and vulvodynia occur far more frequently in perimenopause and menopausal women, estrogen deficiency may be a potential common etiologic mechanism for these 2 entities. Estrogen receptors have been identified in both the tongue salivary glands and the vaginal mucosa.[43] Some reports have shown hormone replacement therapy in postmenopausal patients with oral discomfort to be useful[44,45] whereas others have not seen significant improvement in the symptom presentation utilizing this approach.[46]

Steroid dysregulation
Recently, Woda and colleagues[47] have suggested a potential association of BMS presentation with an alteration of gonadal, adrenal and neuroactive steroid levels. They suggested that prolonged anxiety or stress might result in a dysregulation and reduction of adrenal steroid production. A comparative study of BMS patients and controls demonstrated an increase in anxiety scores as well as salivary cortisol levels in the BMS population.[48] An increased level of salivary cortisol has also been observed in patients with chronic stress.[49] This over-production of cortisol over a prolonged period could potentially lead to cortisol depletion or hypocortisolism. It has been demonstrated that both low levels and high levels of cortisol may be damaging to neural tissues.[50]

Neuropathic Considerations

Peripheral small-fiber neuropathy
Damage to peripheral small nerve fibers can result in clinical presentations often described as burning, tingling, and numb. Grushka[16] showed that BMS patients tend to have a decreased tolerance to a painful heat stimulus at the tip of the tongue compared with healthy control subjects. Small nerve fiber neuropathy has been shown along with a significant reduction in density of small fibers in the areas of pain in BMS populations.[51,52] Forssell and colleagues[53] also demonstrated an atypical sensory threshold in the tongue in 76% of 46 BMS patients examined by quantitative sensory testing. Lauria[54] performed superficial biopsies of the lateral aspect of the anterior two-thirds of the tongue in 12 confirmed BMS patients and found a significant loss of epithelial and subpapillary nerve fibers in these areas.

Enhanced transient receptor potential vanilloid 1 receptors
The transient receptor potential (TRP) protein group consists of voltage-independent calcium-permeable channels. These channels are responsible for thermal sensations ranging from extreme cold to extreme heat.[55] The TRP vanilloid 1 (TRPV1) receptor, also known as the capsaicin receptor, is activated by noxious heat and capsaicin.[56] Yilmaz and colleagues[52] demonstrated an up-regulation of TRPV1 fibers in BMS subjects compared with controls. TRPV1 up-regulation has also been noted with rectal hypersensitivity and vulvodynia.[57,58]

Sensory purinergic receptor activity
The purinergic receptors have been previously categorized into 2 major classes: the P1 receptors that are endogenously activated by adenosine and the P2 receptors that are activated by ATP.[59] The P2 receptors are then further divided into 2 groups; the ligand-gated ion channels, known as P2X receptors, and the G-protein–coupled receptors, called P2Y receptors.[60] There are 7 described P2X receptor types, of which 6 are located on primary sensory neurons.[61] Of those 6, the P2X3 receptor is expressed primarily in small neurons of sensory ganglia.[62] A study by Beneng and

colleagues[63] revealed an increase in P2X3 immunoreactive nerve fibers in tongue biopsies taken from BMS patients. They conclude that an increased P2X3 immunoreactivity in the trigeminal sensory system due to an increase in ATP release may play an important, albeit yet to be fully described role, in the development and maintenance of BMS.

Subclinical major trigeminal neuropathy

An intimate relationship between the fifth and seventh cranial nerves is well known. The mucosa of the tongue is innervated by both the facial nerve via the chorda tympani and the trigeminal nerve via the lingual branch. These 2 structures share a common pathway en route to the tongue. Fibers of the lingual nerve then terminate in the taste buds in fungiform papillae. The chorda tympani nerve provides innervation to the taste pores of the taste buds in these same papillae. Wang and colleagues[64] suggested an electrophysiologic interaction between these 2 nerves, designed to modulate the taste function of the chorda tympani nerve. Damage to either nerve may influence the other intact nerve as seen in other models of neuropathic pain.[65] Damage may be due to occasional minor injuries incurred by consuming excessively hot food or beverage or by common dental procedures or anesthetic injections. It has been suggested that approximately 20% to 25% of BMS presentations are resultant from some form of subclinical lingual, mandibular, or trigeminal system pathology that may be revealed with a comprehensive neurophysiologic examination. Review of the masseter reflex and blink reflex and its habituation in primary BMS patients has demonstrated significant abnormalities in the large fibers of the trigeminal nerve distribution.[53,66]

Central pain related to deficient dopaminergic inhibition

PET studies have shown a decrease in striatal endogenous dopamine levels and a resultant deficiency in dopamine mediated descending pain modulation in the trigeminal brainstem complex in BMS subjects.[67,68] These PET findings are similar to those found in early Parkinson disease.[69] A case report using pramipexol, a known dopaminergic agonist used in the treatment of Parkinson disease, saw complete remission of BMS in a 68-year-old woman.[70] The investigators admitted their results were anecdotal and possibly due to placebo effect and/or simply coincidental. Ultimately, this outcome needs to be confirmed by more robust studies. Overall, based on imaging studies and sensory testing results, it may be suggested that deficient descending inhibition of pain by means of the striatal dopamine loop may present a risk factor for the development of chronic neuropathic oral and facial pains including BMS.[71]

DIAGNOSTIC AND INVESTIGATIVE STRATEGIES
History

A diagnosis of BMS is considered to be one of exclusion of all secondary factors. A comprehensive medical and dental history, including a complete review of current medications, along with an exhaustive review of systems is essential for establishing a definitive diagnosis. Patients' descriptions of their present concern, including a history of their symptom onset and progression and any associated symptoms, and a description of any previous and current treatments should be included. The intensity of the presenting pain should be measured using appropriate scales. The character and distribution of their pain should to be assessed. Factors that worsen as well as those that lessen their pain are important to include in the history. Patients should be queried as to any history of previous upper respiratory tract infections, middle ear disease, or surgery that may have damaged the chorda tympani nerve. A patient's dietary habits as well as the use of oral care products should be investigated. An appropriate psychosocial history should also be considered as a component of the comprehensive history to determine the presence or status of any past or current psychosocial stressors.

Physical Examination

The clinical examination is intended to identify or rule out factors that may contribute to a patient's concern. The extraoral examination should include a general inspection of the head, face, and neck for evidence of trauma, tumors, or previous radiation therapy. The neck should be evaluated for evidence of goiter, lymphadenopathy, or lymphadenitis. The temporomandibular joint complexes as well as the muscles of mastication should be appropriately palpated and jaw function assessed. Neurologic screening, including a cranial nerve assessment, is recommended. The oral cavity should be inspected to assess the health of the mucosa, periodontium, and dentition. Any dental prosthetic device should be thoroughly evaluated.

Laboratory Studies

The need for laboratory studies should be guided by the results of the history and physical examination. When all clinical findings are within normal limitations, a more comprehensive approach to testing is suggested.
Recommended studies include

- Complete blood cell count with differential
- Fasting blood glucose
- Hemoglobin A_{1c}
- Thyroid function (T3/T4)
- Serum iron
- Ferritin
- Total IgE
- Vitamin B_6, vitamin B_{12}, and vitamin D
- Serum antinuclear antibodies
- Anti-Sjögren's-syndrome-related antigen A and Anti-Sjögren's-syndrome-related antigen B (SSA/Ro and SSB/La)
- Erythrocyte sedimentation rate
- Serum antibodies to *Helicobacter pylori* and oral candida
- Viral and bacterial swabs

Adjunctive Testing

Imaging of the brain and brainstem via CT or MRI is suggested if pain presentation seems atypical of a normal presentation. This may include findings of sensory and/or motor disturbances, autonomic changes, or any other evidence suggestive of central nervous system pathology or some type of neurodegenerative process. The status of salivary structures may also be identified on appropriate imaging as well. Allergen patch testing may be useful in some cases. This testing is typically reserved for patients with evidence of a lichenoid-like tissue lesion on visual inspection of the oral cavity. Sialometry is suggested to determine if oral dryness is a key factor. The amount of saliva flow varies from individual to individual and correlates poorly with the subjective report of a dry mouth. Biopsy of the minor salivary glands is needed to definitively diagnose Sjögren syndrome if suspected. Psychometric testing, which may include the SCL-90R, MPI, the Hospital Anxiety and Depression Scale, and the Beck Depression Inventory, may be considered to evaluate the influence of psychological and/or anxiety factors. Evaluation for gastroesophageal reflux may also prove helpful in some patients.

MANAGEMENT STRATEGIES

Management strategies of BMS patients based on significant evidence is lacking. Clinically, it must be determined if the presentation is primary or secondary. If the complaint seems secondary to an identifiable etiologic factor, treatment of the underlying condition(s) most often alleviates the BMS complaint. Most treatment approaches for primary BMS yield limited success.[72] Because many patients with BMS have consulted many health care providers and experienced unsuccessful outcomes, is important to first spend time listening to their concerns and then provide education as to the nature of their syndrome and possible therapeutic strategies.

Behavioral Therapies

BMS patients should be educated as to the potentially detrimental effects of parafunctional habits, such as clenching, bruxism, and tongue habits. The use of oral care products should be scrutinized and amended to avoid the use of products that contain alcohol and those that contain flavoring agents or other known oral irritants.[73,74] Self-regulatory approaches, such as regular exercise, diaphragmatic breathing, maintaining a proper diet and adequate hydration, and intentional relaxation, have been shown beneficial in reducing chronic pain complaints.[75] Cognitive behavioral therapy provided by trained clinicians has also proved beneficial in some instances.[76]

Topical Therapies

Several topical therapies have been recommended and used in the management for BMS. In a randomized placebo-controlled trial, Gremeau-Richard and colleagues[77] reported significant pain reduction using a protocol in which patients were instructed to suck a 1 mg tablet of clonazepam for 3 minutes and then expectorate. A recent randomized pilot study comparing the efficacy of photobiomodulation with low-level laser therapy to topical clonazepam concluded that low-level laser therapy was superior to clonazepam in improving pain perception at 8 weeks after the end of the protocol.[78]

Other topical agents to consider include[79–81]

- 0.15% Benzydamine hydrochloride 3 times per day
- Salivary substitutes
- Topical antifungals
- Topical capsaicin (0.025% cream) or rinsing with Tabasco sauce and water (1:2–4 solution)

Systemic Therapies

Several systemic therapies have been used for BMS, including those traditionally found effective for neuropathic pain conditions. A recent meta-analysis reviewing the efficacy of clonazepam used both as a topical agent and taken systemically reported positive therapeutic outcomes.[82] Most systematic reviews to date provide little in the way of consistent guidance for systemic therapies for BMS.

Some suggested systemic agents to consider include[79,81,83]

- α-Lipoic acid, 600 mg per day for 2 months
- Clonazepam, 0.5 mg per day at bedtime
- Gabapentin, 100 mg to 300 mg up to 3 times per day
- Pregabalin, 25 mg to 75 mg up to 3 times per day
- Serotonin/norepinephrine reuptake inhibitor: sertraline, 50 mg per day; paroxetine, 20 mg per day; or duloxetine 30 mg to 60 mg per day

- Salivary stimulant: pilocarpine, 5 mg to 10 mg 3 times per day, or cevimeline, 30 mg 3 times per day
- Tricyclic antidepressant (TCA): amitriptyline, 25 mg to 100 mg per day at bedtime, or nortriptyline, 10 to 75 mg per day at bedtime

A recent case series (6 BMS patients) studied the effect of botulinum toxin A injected intradermally (16 total units) into the tongue and lower lip.[84] All 6 patients in this limited trial reported sustained pain relief, lasting up to 20 weeks for 1 individual.

SUMMARY

BMS is a relatively common and mostly chronic intraoral pain syndrome that remains a diagnostic and treatment challenge to both health care providers and patients suffering with this entity. One of the most important things a practitioner can do is for BMS patients is to validate their story and provide reassurance through education. Patients must be made aware that this syndrome is most likely of multifactorial etiologies involving multiple physiologic processes. They must understand that, currently, there is no cure for BMS and that current therapies are targeted more toward symptom control. Because most patients suffering from BMS have previously consulted with several clinicians, it is paramount that the process of symptom management begins with a comprehensive diagnostic work-up. Using a multimodal and multidisciplinary approach, including medical and psychosocial therapy, provides the best opportunity for symptom relief in patients with BMS. Ultimately, well-designed translational research is needed for this syndrome.

REFERENCES

1. Grushka M, Epstein JB, Gorsky M. Burning mouth syndrome. Am Fam Physician 2002;65(4):615–20.
2. das Neves de Araujo Lima E, Barbosa NG, Dos Santos AC, et al. Comparative analysis of psychological, hormonal, and genetic factors between burning mouth syndrome and secondary oral burning. Pain Med 2016;17(9):1602–11.
3. Pain AAoO. Diagnosis and management of TMDs. In: De Leeuw RKG, editor. Orofacial pain: guidelines for assessment, diagnosis, and management. 5th edition. Chicago: Quintessence; 2013. p. 95–6.
4. Merskey HBN. Descriptions of chronic pain syndromes and definitions of pain terms. Classification of chronic pain. 2nd edition. Seattle (WA): IASP Press; 1994. p. 74–5.
5. Headache Classification Committee of the International Headache Society (IHS). The international classification of headache disorders, 3rd edition (beta version). Cephalalgia 2013;33(9):629–808.
6. Drage LA, Rogers RS 3rd. Burning mouth syndrome. Dermatol Clin 2003;21(1): 135–45.
7. Scala A, Checchi L, Montevecchi M, et al. Update on burning mouth syndrome: overview and patient management. Crit Rev Oral Biol Med 2003;14(4):275–91.
8. Lamey PJ. Burning mouth syndrome. Dermatol Clin 1996;14(2):339–54.
9. Lamey PJ, Lewis MA. Oral medicine in practice: orofacial pain. Br Dent J 1989; 167(11):384–9.
10. Jaaskelainen SK. Pathophysiology of primary burning mouth syndrome. Clin Neurophysiol 2012;123(1):71–7.
11. Coculescu EC, Tovaru S, Coculescu BI. Epidemiological and etiological aspects of burning mouth syndrome. J Med Life 2014;7(3):305–9.

12. Kohorst JJ, Bruce AJ, Torgerson RR, et al. The prevalence of burning mouth syndrome: a population-based study. Br J Dermatol 2015;172(6):1654–6.
13. Forssell H, Jaaskelainen S, List T, et al. An update on pathophysiological mechanisms related to idiopathic oro-facial pain conditions with implications for management. J Oral Rehabil 2015;42(4):300–22.
14. Lopez-Jornet P, Camacho-Alonso F, Andujar-Mateos P, et al. Burning mouth syndrome: an update. Med Oral Patol Oral Cir Bucal 2010;15(4):e562–8.
15. Grinspan D, Fernandez Blanco G, Allevato MA, et al. Burning mouth syndrome. Int J Dermatol 1995;34(7):483–7.
16. Grushka M. Clinical features of burning mouth syndrome. Oral Surg Oral Med Oral Pathol 1987;63(1):30–6.
17. Tatullo M, Marrelli M, Scacco S, et al. Relationship between oxidative stress and "burning mouth syndrome" in female patients: a scientific hypothesis. Eur Rev Med Pharmacol Sci 2012;16(9):1218–21.
18. Gurvits GE, Tan A. Burning mouth syndrome. World J Gastroenterol 2013;19(5): 665–72.
19. Bergdahl M, Bergdahl J. Burning mouth syndrome: prevalence and associated factors. J Oral Pathol Med 1999;28(8):350–4.
20. Woda A, Navez ML, Picard P, et al. A possible therapeutic solution for stomatodynia (burning mouth syndrome). J Orofac Pain 1998;12(4):272–8.
21. Gaitonde P, Rostron J, Longman L, et al. Burning mouth syndrome and vulvodynia coexisting in the same patient: a case report. Dent Update 2002;29(2):75–6.
22. Patton LL, Siegel MA, Benoliel R, et al. Management of burning mouth syndrome: systematic review and management recommendations. Oral Surg Oral Med Oral Pathol Oral Radiol Endod 2007;103(Suppl):S39.e1-13.
23. Poon R, Su N, Ching V, et al. Reduction in unstimulated salivary flow rate in burning mouth syndrome. Br Dent J 2014;217(7):E14.
24. Spadari F, Venesia P, Azzi L, et al. Low basal salivary flow and burning mouth syndrome: new evidence in this enigmatic pathology. J Oral Pathol Med 2015;44(3): 229–33.
25. Forssell H, Teerijoki-Oksa T, Kotiranta U, et al. Pain and pain behavior in burning mouth syndrome: a pain diary study. J Orofac Pain 2012;26(2):117–25.
26. Kenchadze R, Iverieli M, Okribelashvili N, et al. The psychological aspects of burning mouth syndrome. Georgian Med News 2011;(194):24–8.
27. de Souza FT, Teixeira AL, Amaral TM, et al. Psychiatric disorders in burning mouth syndrome. J Psychosom Res 2012;72(2):142–6.
28. Carlson CR, Miller CS, Reid KI. Psychosocial profiles of patients with burning mouth syndrome. J Orofac Pain 2000;14(1):59–64.
29. Osaki T, Yoneda K, Yamamoto T, et al. Candidiasis may induce glossodynia without objective manifestation. Am J Med Sci 2000;319(2):100–5.
30. Ching V, Grushka M, Darling M, et al. Increased prevalence of geographic tongue in burning mouth complaints: a retrospective study. Oral Surg Oral Med Oral Pathol Oral Radiol 2012;114(4):444–8.
31. Lamey PJ, Hammond A, Allam BF, et al. Vitamin status of patients with burning mouth syndrome and the response to replacement therapy. Br Dent J 1986; 160(3):81–4.
32. Cho GS, Han MW, Lee B, et al. Zinc deficiency may be a cause of burning mouth syndrome as zinc replacement therapy has therapeutic effects. J Oral Pathol Med 2010;39(9):722–7.
33. Grushka M, Sessle BJ. Burning mouth syndrome. Dent Clin North Am 1991;35(1): 171–84.

34. Suarez P, Clark GT. Burning mouth syndrome: an update on diagnosis and treatment methods. J Calif Dent Assoc 2006;34(8):611–22.
35. Savino LB, Haushalter NM. Lisinopril-induced "scalded mouth syndrome". Ann Pharmacother 1992;26(11):1381–2.
36. Brown RS, Krakow AM, Douglas T, et al. "Scalded mouth syndrome" caused by angiotensin converting enzyme inhibitors: two case reports. Oral Surg Oral Med Oral Pathol Oral Radiol Endod 1997;83(6):665–7.
37. Bartoshuk LM, Snyder DJ, Grushka M, et al. Taste damage: previously unsuspected consequences. Chem Senses 2005;30(Suppl 1):i218–9.
38. Bartoshuk LMCA, Duffy VB, Gruhska M, et al. Oral phantoms: evidence for central inhibition produced by taste. Chem Senses 2002;27:A52.
39. Schobel N, Kyereme J, Minovi A, et al. Sweet taste and chorda tympani transection alter capsaicin-induced lingual pain perception in adult human subjects. Physiol Behav 2012;107(3):368–73.
40. Bartoshuk LM, Duffy VB, Miller IJ. PTC/PROP tasting: anatomy, psychophysics, and sex effects. Physiol Behav 1994;56(6):1165–71.
41. Grushka M, Epstein JB, Gorsky M. Burning mouth syndrome and other oral sensory disorders: a unifying hypothesis. Pain Res Manag 2003;8(3):133–5.
42. Gao J, Chen L, Zhou J, et al. A case-control study on etiological factors involved in patients with burning mouth syndrome. J Oral Pathol Med 2009;38(1):24–8.
43. Leimola-Virtanen R, Salo T, Toikkanen S, et al. Expression of estrogen receptor (ER) in oral mucosa and salivary glands. Maturitas 2000;36(2):131–7.
44. Forabosco A, Criscuolo M, Coukos G, et al. Efficacy of hormone replacement therapy in postmenopausal women with oral discomfort. Oral Surg Oral Med Oral Pathol 1992;73(5):570–4.
45. Wardrop RW, Hailes J, Burger H, et al. Oral discomfort at menopause. Oral Surg Oral Med Oral Pathol 1989;67(5):535–40.
46. Meurman JH, Tarkkila L, Tiitinen A. The menopause and oral health. Maturitas 2009;63(1):56–62.
47. Woda A, Dao T, Gremeau-Richard C. Steroid dysregulation and stomatodynia (burning mouth syndrome). J Orofac Pain 2009;23(3):202–10.
48. Amenabar JM, Pawlowski J, Hilgert JB, et al. Anxiety and salivary cortisol levels in patients with burning mouth syndrome: case-control study. Oral Surg Oral Med Oral Pathol Oral Radiol Endod 2008;105(4):460–5.
49. Heuser I, Lammers CH. Stress and the brain. Neurobiol Aging 2003;24(Suppl 1):S69–76 [discussion: S81–2].
50. Kaufer D, Ogle WO, Pincus ZS, et al. Restructuring the neuronal stress response with anti-glucocorticoid gene delivery. Nat Neurosci 2004;7(9):947–53.
51. de Tommaso M, Lavolpe V, Di Venere D, et al. A case of unilateral burning mouth syndrome of neuropathic origin. Headache 2011;51(3):441–3.
52. Yilmaz Z, Renton T, Yiangou Y, et al. Burning mouth syndrome as a trigeminal small fibre neuropathy: increased heat and capsaicin receptor TRPV1 in nerve fibres correlates with pain score. J Clin Neurosci 2007;14(9):864–71.
53. Forssell H, Jaaskelainen S, Tenovuo O, et al. Sensory dysfunction in burning mouth syndrome. Pain 2002;99(1–2):41–7.
54. Lauria G. Small fibre neuropathies. Curr Opin Neurol 2005;18(5):591–7.
55. Jordt SE, McKemy DD, Julius D. Lessons from peppers and peppermint: the molecular logic of thermosensation. Curr Opin Neurobiol 2003;13(4):487–92.
56. Caterina MJ, Schumacher MA, Tominaga M, et al. The capsaicin receptor: a heat-activated ion channel in the pain pathway. Nature 1997;389(6653):816–24.

57. Chan CL, Facer P, Davis JB, et al. Sensory fibres expressing capsaicin receptor TRPV1 in patients with rectal hypersensitivity and faecal urgency. Lancet 2003; 361(9355):385–91.

58. Tympanidis P, Casula MA, Yiangou Y, et al. Increased vanilloid receptor VR1 innervation in vulvodynia. Eur J Pain 2004;8(2):129–33.

59. Burnstock G. Purinergic nerves and receptors. Prog Biochem Pharmacol 1980; 16:141–54.

60. Ralevic V, Burnstock G. Receptors for purines and pyrimidines. Pharmacol Rev 1998;50(3):413–92.

61. Cockayne DA, Dunn PM, Zhong Y, et al. P2X2 knockout mice and P2X2/P2X3 double knockout mice reveal a role for the P2X2 receptor subunit in mediating multiple sensory effects of ATP. J Physiol 2005;567(Pt 2):621–39.

62. Chen CC, Akopian AN, Sivilotti L, et al. A P2X purinoceptor expressed by a subset of sensory neurons. Nature 1995;377(6548):428–31.

63. Beneng K, Yilmaz Z, Yiangou Y, et al. Sensory purinergic receptor P2X3 is elevated in burning mouth syndrome. Int J Oral Maxillofac Surg 2010;39(8): 815–9.

64. Wang Y, Erickson RP, Simon SA. Modulation of rat chorda tympani nerve activity by lingual nerve stimulation. J Neurophysiol 1995;73(4):1468–83.

65. Shortland PJ, Baytug B, Krzyzanowska A, et al. ATF3 expression in L4 dorsal root ganglion neurons after L5 spinal nerve transection. Eur J Neurosci 2006;23(2): 365–73.

66. Jaaskelainen SK, Forssell H, Tenovuo O. Abnormalities of the blink reflex in burning mouth syndrome. Pain 1997;73(3):455–60.

67. Jaaskelainen SK, Rinne JO, Forssell H, et al. Role of the dopaminergic system in chronic pain – a fluorodopa-PET study. Pain 2001;90(3):257–60.

68. Hagelberg N, Forssell H, Rinne JO, et al. Striatal dopamine D1 and D2 receptors in burning mouth syndrome. Pain 2003;101(1–2):149–54.

69. Heiss WD, Herholz K. Brain receptor imaging. J Nucl Med 2006;47(2):302–12.

70. Stuginski-Barbosa J, Rodrigues GG, Bigal ME, et al. Burning mouth syndrome responsive to pramipexol. J Headache Pain 2008;9(1):43–5.

71. Jaaskelainen SK, Lindholm P, Valmunen T, et al. Variation in the dopamine D2 receptor gene plays a key role in human pain and its modulation by transcranial magnetic stimulation. Pain 2014;155(10):2180–7.

72. Sardella A, Lodi G, Demarosi F, et al. Burning mouth syndrome: a retrospective study investigating spontaneous remission and response to treatments. Oral Dis 2006;12(2):152–5.

73. Endo H, Rees TD. Cinnamon products as a possible etiologic factor in orofacial granulomatosis. Med Oral Patol Oral Cir Bucal 2007;12(6):E440–4.

74. Minor JS, Epstein JB. Burning mouth syndrome and secondary oral burning. Otolaryngol Clin North Am 2011;44(1):205–19, vii.

75. Sauer SE, Burris JL, Carlson CR. New directions in the management of chronic pain: self-regulation theory as a model for integrative clinical psychology practice. Clin Psychol Rev 2010;30(6):805–14.

76. Bergdahl J, Anneroth G, Perris H. Cognitive therapy in the treatment of patients with resistant burning mouth syndrome: a controlled study. J Oral Pathol Med 1995;24(5):213–5.

77. Gremeau-Richard C, Woda A, Navez ML, et al. Topical clonazepam in stomatodynia: a randomised placebo-controlled study. Pain 2004;108(1–2):51–7.

78. Arduino PG, Cafaro A, Garrone M, et al. A randomized pilot study to assess the safety and the value of low-level laser therapy versus clonazepam in patients with burning mouth syndrome. Lasers Med Sci 2016;31(4):811–6.
79. Aravindhan R, Vidyalakshmi S, Kumar MS, et al. Burning mouth syndrome: a review on its diagnostic and therapeutic approach. J Pharm Bioallied Sci 2014; 6(Suppl 1):S21–5.
80. Coculescu EC, Radu A, Coculescu BI. Burning mouth syndrome: a review on diagnosis and treatment. J Med Life 2014;7(4):512–5.
81. Miziara I, Chagury A, Vargas C, et al. Therapeutic options in idiopathic burning mouth syndrome: literature review. Int Arch Otorhinolaryngol 2015;19(1):86–9.
82. Cui Y, Xu H, Chen F, et al. Efficacy evaluation of clonazepam for symptom remission in burning mouth syndrome: a meta-analysis. Oral Dis 2015. https://doi.org/10.1111/odi.12422.
83. Grushka M, Epstein J, Mott A. An open-label, dose escalation pilot study of the effect of clonazepam in burning mouth syndrome. Oral Surg Oral Med Oral Pathol Oral Radiol Endod 1998;86(5):557–61.
84. Restivo DA, Lauria G, Marchese-Ragona R, et al. Botulinum toxin for burning mouth syndrome. Ann Intern Med 2017;166(10):762–3.

Painful Oral Lesions

Istvan A. Hargitai, DDS, MS*

KEYWORDS

- Vesiculoerosive • Vesiculobullous • Aphthous ulcer • Herpes labialis

KEY POINTS

- Oral lesions generally fall into the category of either being neoplastic, inflammatory, reactive, or developmental.
- Painful oral vesiculoerosive diseases (OVD) discussed here are reactions to an autoimmune or a viral pathosis with a secondary inflammatory component.
- First-line treatment of autoimmune-related OVD are topical or systemic corticosteroids. Extraoral lesions need referral to an appropriate physician.
- For optimal treatment of herpetic oral lesions, antiviral medications should be instituted as soon as possible within the first day or 2.

Pain is a powerful motivator to seek medical or dental care. When that pain is combined with a visible, physical lesion or abnormality, health care providers should expect these patients to present with a great deal of concern and anxiety about their condition. Dental practitioners should be well-versed in pain conditions that occur outside of the dentition and periodontium. Oral health care providers are key to the identification and management of the more common painful oral lesions that patients may present with. In addition to the pain and anxiety concerning oral lesions, there is further concern that these ailments would interfere with mastication, nutritional intake and speech.

In general, lesions can be classified via the NIRD acronym: neoplastic, inflammatory, reactive, and developmental. Even if the clinical diagnosis is elusive, by way of history and clinical examination, the clinician may be able to at least classify the lesion into one of the above categories. For example, there is an erythematous lesion in the soft tissues adjacent to tooth no. 30. History includes placement of a large amalgam restoration adjacent to the lesion a short time before the lesion was noticed. Cognitively, the clinician should at least consider that the lesion may represent a reactive process.

The following additional information can help further subdivide an oral lesion into a clinical differential diagnosis:

- Location: Where inside the oral cavity is the lesion? Besides the presence of oral lesion(s), are there any lesions present at other body locations? If yes, the disease entity can be part of a wider systemic or dermatologic condition.

Disclosure: The author has nothing to disclose.
Naval Postgraduate Dental School, Bethesda, MD, USA
* 8955 Wood Road, Bethesda, MD 20889-5628.
E-mail address: hargitai70@hotmail.com

Dent Clin N Am 62 (2018) 597–609
https://doi.org/10.1016/j.cden.2018.06.002
0011-8532/18/Published by Elsevier Inc.

dental.theclinics.com

- How many? Is the oral lesion single or multiple? The chancre associated with primary syphilis is a single lesion at the site of viral inoculation. Lesions of condyloma acuminatum associated with human papilloma virus are multiple.
- How long has the lesion(s) been there? This will help determine if the lesion is an acute process or a chronic state.
- Has this ever happened before? This will help determine if it is a primary event or part of a condition whereby recurrence is known to happen.
- Color: White, red, mixed, purple, or pigmented. For example, hemangiomas are purple or red in color and not white.

The above data also make for useful information to include in the patient record.

ORAL VESICULOEROSIVE DISEASES

Oral vesiculoerosive diseases (OVD) are a group of conditions that effect mucocutaneous tissues to include the oral cavity. They present with smaller vesicles or larger bullae (ie, blisters) that can rupture to leave painful denuded mucosa or ulcers. The most relevant of the OVD are those that have a proposed autoimmune or allergen-related cause to their pathophysiology. Several relatively common OVDs are presented followed by their collective treatment, because their management is often similar. Treatments unique to a given condition are addressed within their respective sections.

Lichen Planus

Lichen planus (LP) is a chronic disease affecting the skin and/or mucous membranes. Dermal LP is often self-limiting. The skin lesions associated with LP present as the 4 P's: pruritic, polygonal, purple papules. Oral lichen planus (OLP) may be symptomatic or asymptomatic. Symptomatic OLP may be quite painful if not outright debilitating. In the worst cases, speech and nutrition are often difficult secondary to the pain. Most commonly, OLP is unaccompanied by LP at other sites.

Relative to the other OVD, OLP is rather common. A review of population studies puts the overall prevalence at 1.27% (0.96% in men, 1.57% in women).[1] Two-thirds of cases are found in women with the average age at diagnosis in the late 50s, with an age range of 11 to 94.[1-4] OLP affects individuals of all races, but reports are more frequent from India.[1]

Clinical features of OLP are that of a flat, erythematous base that is interlaced with raised white lines (Wickham striae) or patches. Lesions are often symmetric and diffuse. By far the most affected oral site is the buccal mucosa with other common sites being the tongue, gingiva, and vestibule.[2,3,5] When OLP affects the gingiva, in those cases it is often the only site. When the gingiva becomes involved, it may present with erythema, ulceration, and bleeding. The outer layer of the gingiva may separate and slough off, leaving behind a raw, red, painful surface. The sloughing process is referred to as a desquamative gingivitis. However, other OVDs such as pemphigus vulgaris (PV) and mucous membrane pemphigoid (MMP) may also present as such and should be differentiated from OLP.

Although most cases of OLP are asymptomatic, when symptoms are present, pain is the most common feature (reported 27%–43%) but can also be accompanied by reports of xerostomia, mucosal roughness, and dysgeusia.[2,3] Symptoms tend to wax and wane over time. Quiescent periods may be interrupted by acute exacerbations of pain. Clinical subtypes of OLP are based on appearance and can include the common reticular form of OLP (**Fig. 1**) and also the more painful form called erosive lichen planus (ELP).[6] Less common are the plaque, bullous, and papular subtypes.[7] The clinical subtype can progress from a less symptomatic variety (reticular OLP) to a more painful variety (ELP) and vice versa. Over time, 65% of the cases have the

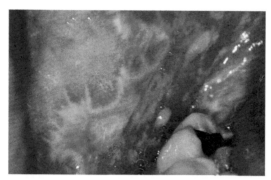

Fig. 1. The reticular form of OLP in the buccal mucosa of a Caucasian man. (*Courtesy of* Istvan A. Hargitai, DDS, MS, Bethesda, MD.)

same subtype of OLP seen at baseline or the disease had progressed to a more severe form, whereas in 35% percent of cases, the condition changed to a less severe form.[4] There is a small but notable malignant transformation rate of OLP to squamous cell carcinoma (SCC). This transformation rate has been estimated to occur between 1% and 3% of cases, particularly with the ELP subtype.[6,8]

Regarding diagnosis, although the reticular form of OLP is quite characteristic of the condition, the other subtypes can be confused with any of the other OVDs. In the case of ELP at an isolated site, it may even mimic the appearance of SCC. However, ELP is typically painful, whereas SCC is often not unless neural invasion has occurred. Regardless of appearance, any oral lesion that does not resolve in 2 weeks should undergo biopsy and histologic examination. An adequate specimen of about 8 mm across in a representative area of the lesion, ideally with a sample of normal tissue, should be obtained and fixed in 10% formalin. At the pathology laboratory, the specimen is stained with hematoxylin and eosin (H&E) for histologic examination. Classic OLP histologically may display saw-tooth rete pegs with an underlying dense, band-like infiltrate of lymphocytes within the fibrous connective tissue.

Prognosis in OLP is that the lesions may regress or progress, and thus, it is a chronic condition. Once the entity is correctly identified, flares of pain may be managed effectively with corticosteroids. The ELP subtype should be monitored minimally at 6- to 12-month intervals in order to observe the appearance of the lesions. Any change in character that arouses suspicion for dysplasia or malignant transformation should be rebiopsied. Clinical photographs for the record can be used to compare the lesions from one time period to the next. The monitoring for malignant transformation may readily coincide with regularly scheduled dental checkups and hygiene appointments.

Treatment of OLP primarily revolves around corticosteroids and is discussed later. As an alternative, levamisole and tacrolimus have been used with some success but with limited studies.[9]

Pemphigus Vulgaris

PV is a rare but potentially serious mucocutaneous vesiculobullous disease. It is one of 6 forms of pemphigus to include the following: (1) PV, (2) pemphigus vegetans, (3) immunoglobulin A pemphigus, (4) pemphigus foliaceous, (5) pemphigus erythematosus, and (6) paraneoplastic pemphigus.[10] The first 3 may manifest with oral lesions. This article primarily focuses on PV. Of note, with paraneoplastic pemphigus is its association with several neoplasms, the most common being non-Hodgkin lymphoma.[11] The incidence of PV is 0.1 to 0.5 per 100,000 people, has a slight female predilection, and although it may affect individuals of any age, most cases present between ages 40 to 60 years, and the condition is most notable in those individuals of Mediterranean descent.[12]

PV affects the skin and the oral mucosa. Skin involvement can include the esophagus, genitalia, and conjunctival mucosa. The dental professional is in the unique position to be the first to notice the lesions of PV, because 80% of PV cases present with oral lesions before the onset of skin lesions.[12] Oral presentation provides an opportunity for early detection and identification of PV. Should skin lesions of PV subsequently occur, the patient will be able to report this history to their primary care manager, and thus, treatment can be initiated rapidly. Before the advent of corticosteroids, dermal sloughing led to fluid loss and infection, and up until the mid-twentieth century, its mortality rate approached 90%.[12]

Clinically, oral PV may appear on the buccal mucosa, palate, and gingiva (**Fig. 2**). Rubbing the gingiva with gauze or the back end of a dental instrument can induce a bulla. This bulla is a positive Nikolsky sign. The lesions initially present as bullae and then quickly rupture into painful ulcers, which is the cardinal presenting sign and symptom. Precipitating factors of PV are thought to include genetic predisposition, stress, diet, medication, or malignancy.[13] Implicated medications include aspirin, nonsteroidal anti-inflammatory drugs, cephalosporins, and angiotensin-converting enzyme inhibitors.[10] The most commonly held cause of PV is thought to involve autoantibodies directed at adhesion molecules against dermal and mucosal cells. Autoantibodies specifically target the anchoring elements desmoglein 1 (Dsg1) and 3 (Dsg3) in squamous cells.[12] Dsg3 is more prevalent in oral mucosa, while the skin features both Dsg1 and Dsg3.

A diagnosis can be obtained via soft tissue biopsy as described under the LP heading for H&E staining. A second biopsy of the represented area, or splitting a larger biopsy specimen in half to be fixed in Michel's solution, is used for the purpose of direct immunofluorescence (DIF) to observe the location of antibodies directed against immunoglobulin and complement deposits. With DIF, the cell surfaces fluoresce in a "fishnet pattern." Both stains show an "intraepithelial split" within the surface cells of the epithelium or mucosa superficial to the basement membrane and its basal cells. These basal cells with the clefted area above give the basal cell layer a "row of tombstones" appearance. The cells of the spinous layer are acantholytic, and isolated cells can become circular in shape, the so-called Tzanck cell. In some cases, a sample of the patient's blood is obtained for serum indirect immunofluorescence (IIF) to better define prognosis and therapy.[12]

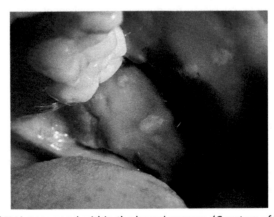

Fig. 2. Lesions of PV interspersed within the buccal mucosa. (*Courtesy of* Istvan A. Hargitai, DDS, MS, Bethesda, MD.)

Consulting with a dermatologist is recommended with the presence of skin lesions. The cornerstone of PV management is corticosteroids. However, corticosteroids alone do not always bring PV into remission, and the addition of immunosuppressive drugs is often needed. Before the age of corticosteroids, PV was life threatening. The steroid-sparing alternatives to consider as first line drugs are mycophenolate and azathioprine.[14]

Mucous Membrane Pemphigoid

MMP, formerly known cicatricial pemphigoid, benign mucous membrane pemphigoid, or just simply pemphigoid, is primarily an affliction of the elderly. The incidence of MMP is approximately 1.3 to 2.0 per million per year.[15–17] There appears to be no ethnic predilection for this condition. However, there are gender and age differences. Women are affected almost 2:1 over men. Peak incidence occurs in older individuals typically between the ages of 60 and 65.[15] Like PV, the cause of MMP is autoimmune.

MMP occurs as skin or mucous membrane fluid-filled vesicles or bullae that rupture into painful ulcers or larger segments of sloughing, leaving sensitive, denuded patches. The lesions of MMP tend to be redder than those of PV. Affected oral sites include the gingiva, buccal mucosa, and palate.[16] Other oral sites are much less involved. The lesions need up to 2 weeks to heal. Like PV, when the sloughing involves the gingiva, it is again termed a desquamative gingivitis. Another repeat feature to PV is a positive Nikolsky sign (**Fig. 3**). The top 2 sites affected by MMP are the oral mucosa (85%) and the conjunctiva of the eyes (65%–80%).[15] The propensity for ocular lesions can progress to blindness. Early consultation with an ophthalmologist is recommended as soon as possible. The conjunctiva scar and contract down, forming an adhesion called a symblepharon. When lesions occur on the skin, they often heal with a scar. Definitive diagnosis of MMP is by biopsy using either H&E or DIF staining. The histopathologic appearance is a characteristic "subepithelial split," where the entire epithelial surface separates from its underlying connective tissue layer. DIF features of MMP show a linear band of fluorescence at the basement membrane layer. IIF is less helpful in diagnosis in MMP compared with PV or bullous pemphigoid.[16]

Initial treatment of MMP with isolated oral involvement is with corticosteroids in topical, rinse, or systemic forms.[16] More severe cases, or those with ocular involvement, may require combination treatment with either cyclosporine, azathioprine, or

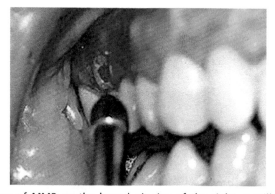

Fig. 3. Oral lesions of MMP on the buccal gingiva of the right, maxillary sextant. Note that the air-water syringe is pointing to a ruptured bulla that was induced by rubbing the lesion representing a positive Nikolsky sign. (*Courtesy of* Istvan A. Hargitai, DDS, MS, Bethesda, MD.)

cyclophosphamide.[17] An emerging treatment of recalcitrant cases of MMP, other OVD, and certain leukemias is the monoclonal antibody rituximab given intravenously.[18] Referral to an ophthalmologist is necessary for the special considerations of ocular lesion treatment.

Erythema Multiforme

Erythema multiforme (EM) represents an unusual reaction to a drug or an infectious agent that is different from typical allergic reactions. In its more severe from, EM is a part of Stevens-Johnson syndrome (SJS) and toxic epidermal necrolysis (TEN), which are potentially life-threatening conditions.[19] A wide array of medications have been implicated with EM to include sulfa drugs, antibiotics, nonsteroidal anti-inflammatory drugs, and acetaminophen. Infectious agents that have been reported to correlate with the disease include herpes simplex virus (HSV) infections, candidal fungal infections, mycoplasma and mycobacterium species, as well as others.[20,21] Radiation therapy and endocrine triggers have also been reported as initiators.

EM affects people of varying age ranges without a particular gender predilection. The mean age for EM has been reported to be 37 to 43 with an age range of 7 to 78, but is less common past the age of 60. EM is relatively rare, and it is probably more common than SJS and TEN. The incidence of EM is 5 cases per million per year. The incidence of SJS is estimated at 4 to 5 per million per year, whereas the incidence of TEN is reported to be 0.9 to 1.5 per million per year.[19] Suspected causative factors reported to correlate with EM in large cohort studies have been drugs (47%), HSV (30%), and candidosis (20%).[20,21] The causative triggers in SJS and TEN are almost always related to drugs.

EM has an explosive onset compared with other OVD, and pain is the cardinal chief complaint (**Fig. 4**). Thus, onset is acute, and the lesions are multiple. The more commonly affected oral sites are the lips and the buccal mucosa with some floor of the mouth involvement in a smaller percentage of cases.[20] Gingival lesions are notably absent. Intraoral lesions can produce a positive Nikolsky sign. EM often presents with only oral lesions in 47% to 73% of cases.[20,21] When other sites are involved, EM can affect the arms, palms of the hand, and genitalia. When EM involves the hands, it may appear as "target lesions." EM is usually self-limiting with lesions and symptoms present for 10 to 14 days. However, in 37% to 73% of cases, the condition is chronic with episodes of outbreaks and remission.[20,21]

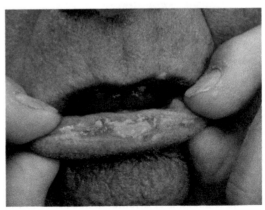

Fig. 4. EM involving the lower lip a Caucasian man in his 6th decade of life. (*Courtesy of* Istvan A. Hargitai, DDS, MS, Bethesda, MD.)

Diagnosis is based on history and biopsy. The clinician should try and correlate a temporal pattern between the pain and lesions and ascertain if there are any new medications or other conditions (viral, fungal, and so forth) that might have occurred at onset or that shortly predated the onset. Histopathology of EM is not pathognomonic as it is with the other OVD. Histologic features can include epithelial layer spongiosis with lymphocytic and eosinophilic infiltrates among other features.

As is the case with the other OVD, EM confined to the oral cavity is initially managed with a short course of low-potency corticosteroids such as topical desonide. More severe cases will need systemic dosing with prednisone. In cases resistant to steroids, the steroid-sparing drug levamisole may be used as monotherapy or in conjunction with prednisone with good response.[22] If HSV or candidosis is suspected, cotreatment with an antiviral such as valacyclovir and an antifungal such as nystatin, respectively, may be used. Cases of EM with skin lesions suggestive of SJS or TEN should be referred to a dermatologist immediately. TEN tends to occur in older individuals. The severe skin sloughing in TEN leads to fluid and electrolyte imbalances analogous to that of severe burn victims. Thus, TEN patients are often managed in hospital burn units.

Recurrent Aphthous Stomatitis

Recurrent aphthous stomatitis (RAS) is referred to as a "canker sore" in lay terms. It is another OVD with an immunopathic pathophysiology with a genetic predisposition. Trauma, certain foods, and stress have all been implicated as triggers. RAS is very common and is reported by 40% of the population.[23] RAS may present in one of 3 clinical forms: minor, major, and herpetiform.[24] Minor RAS is a solitary lesion of less than 6 mm in diameter. Major RAS is a solitary lesion greater than 1 cm in diameter. A mimicker of RAS in appearance includes the solitary lesion of SCC. The difference is that RAS major is exquisitely painful, whereas as SCC generally is not unless neural invasion has occurred. In addition, SCC can occur on any site and may be fixed to underlying connective tissue. Major RAS on the other hand is on freely movable tissues only. Herpetiform RAS presents as multiple lesions, usually one to several millimeters in diameter. The term herpetiform means to imply that it is not due to a herpetic lesion, but rather it refers to its appearance mimicking a cluster of herpetic ulcers.

All forms of RAS present with a lesion or lesions that appear as a gray or tan ulcer with an intense red halo surrounding its border (**Figs. 5** and **6**). The lesion may be covered by a gray pseudomembrane. Vesicles are not observed. A key feature is that RAS lesions occur on unkeratinized, movable tissues only. RAS may affect nearly

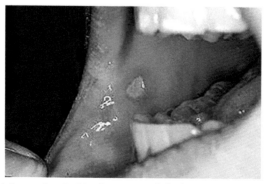

Fig. 5. A minor aphthous ulcer inside the corner of the lips. (*Courtesy of* Istvan A. Hargitai, DDS, MS, Bethesda, MD.)

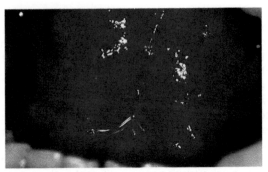

Fig. 6. RAS of the herpetiform variety on the ventral tongue of a young, adult African American man. (*Courtesy of* Istvan A. Hargitai, DDS, MS, Bethesda, MD.)

all surfaces, such as the lips, tongue, buccal mucosa, floor of mouth, and occasionally, the soft palate. The lesions are painful, and depending on lesion size and location, speaking and eating may be difficult and exacerbate the pain. Touching or stretching the lesion may cause the ulcer to break down and result in bleeding. The lesions typically last 10 to 14 days, and the condition is self-limiting even without treatment.[24] A person with RAS will periodically have the condition recur. Recurrence rate varies individual to individual. Diagnosis of RAS can be made by history and clinical presentation, and biopsy is mostly unnecessary unless the case is atypical. The prognosis of RAS is good. Because episodes of ulceration are self-limiting, treatment reduces morbidity. There can be substantial disability if lesions are untreated. A subset of patients will have problems with frequent recurrence. RAS may mimic Behcet syndrome, which is the triad of oral ulcers, genital ulcers, and lesions of the eye.

The management of RAS is focused at reducing pain and morbidity, shrinking the lesions, which also reduces the pain, as well as slightly decreasing the duration of the episode and facilitation of healing. RAS responds very well, and rapidly, to the administration of topical and/or systemic corticosteroids.[23,24] Other treatment can include application of topical local anesthetics such as benzocaine gels. Even better are the 20% benzocaine preparations mixed in with a cellulose compound (Orabase) because it forms a physical barrier over the ulcer to reduce pain from mechanical irritation. The over-the-counter (OTC) topical preparation Zilactin contains 10% benzyl alcohol and forms a protective hydroxypropyl cellulose barrier. In an open-label study, Zilactin reduced RAS pain for a 4-hour period.[25]

MANAGEMENT OF ORAL VESICULOEROSIVE DISEASES

All the OVD have an immunopathic pathophysiology. Modulating inflammatory pathways with immune suppressants that have anti-inflammatory properties attenuate the pain and morbidity associated with these lesions. Corticosteroids remain the first-line medications in the treatment of OVD.[10,13,16,23] Corticosteroids come in a variety of preparations allowing for varied routes of administration. Preparations include pastes/gels, elixirs, systemic medications, and injectable medications (**Table 1**). Topical creams meant for application on the skin should not be used in the mouth.

Topical medicaments are typically used for smaller lesions or lesions confined to an intraoral area that is easily accessible to the patient for application of the medication. A smaller, solitary lesion may be treated with a low-potency triamcinolone alone or compounded in Orabase to enhance contact time. For larger, more painful lesions,

Table 1
Commonly used corticosteroids and their doses with routes of administration in the management of oral vesiculoerosive diseases

Corticosteroid	Dose	Route of Administration
Topical paste or gel		
Triamcinolone	0.25%–1.0%	For mild to moderate cases where lesions are easy to reach by the patient when applying the medicament. Apply 3–4 times daily up to 10 d as needed
Desonide	0.50%	
Fluocinonide	0.05%	
Clobetasol	0.05%	
Elixir		
Dexamethasone	0.5 mg/5 mL	For mild to moderate cases where lesions are too numerous or are inaccessible to topical application. Used as a rinse; in more severe cases, the elixir may be swallowed. Use 3–4 times/d
Prednisolone	5 mg/5 mL	
Systemic		
Prednisone	40–80 mg	For moderate to severe cases, taken once daily early in the morning for 7–10 d. The dose pack is a 6-d course
Methylprednisolone dose pack	4 mg	
Intralesional injection		
Dexamethasone	1 mg	For lesions recalcitrant to topical/systemic dosing. Typically does not need repetition

a medium potency topical such as fluocinonide or desonide may be applied. The most potent topical is clobetasol and is used when the OVD is resistant to less potent topicals. All these medicaments are applied 3 to 4 times daily for a course that typically runs 7 to 14 days or less, depending on symptom or lesion resolution. The role for corticosteroid elixirs comes into play when lesions are too numerous or too difficult to access for the patient and applying topical medications become impractical. Dexamethasone and prednisolone both come in flavorful elixirs that are swished for 1 to 2 minutes and then expectorated. They can be used up to 4 times daily for 7 to 10 days. In more severe cases, the elixir may be swallowed and used as a systemic in those patients unable to swallow pills.

Systemic corticosteroids are used in OVD cases that are large or painful in which significant morbidity is occurring to the point where the condition interferes with eating, talking, or swallowing.[16] The prototypical drug used systemically is prednisone. Based on severity, 40 to 80 mg of prednisone is taken daily for 10 days or so. To minimize some of the side effects that include sleep disturbance, it is advisable to take the dose first thing in the morning to coincide with the natural, diurnal release of the body's own cortisol. In the immune-competent individual, when systemic corticosteroids are used for less than 2 weeks, a steroid taper is not needed. If used greater than 2 weeks, then a taper is needed. Side effects of corticosteroids to both topical and systemic administration are fungal superinfection, particularly to candidal species. Wound healing may be delayed but not so much that treatment needs to be delayed if a biopsy was obtained as part of the diagnostic workup. If an OVD is suspected, particularly if the case is painful, management is initiated. In the case of topical steroids, instruct the patient to avoid direct application at the biopsy site. Consult with a physician would be warranted before initiating systemic corticosteroid therapy in patients with an active infection, latent tuberculosis, uncontrolled diabetes, or those who are immunosuppressed. Painful lesions recalcitrant to topical and/or systemic corticosteroids can often be resolved or greatly improved with an intralesional injection of dexamethasone. The injectable form of dexamethasone is supplied in a strength of 10 mg/mL. Injection of 0.1 mL in the form of a tuberculin syringe, as an example, delivers 1 mg of dexamethasone, which has 25 times the potency of cortisol. Within days to a week, the lesion should decrease markedly in size if not completely resolve.

Lesion resolution is not necessarily a goal of OVD management, except in the case of RAS, where there are lesion-free periods. Although decreasing the size of the lesions does correlate with pain reduction, pain relief can occur even with the lesions still present. It is up to clinical judgment whether a biopsy is required in all OVD cases. The history and appearance of RAS are unique enough that a biopsy is not warranted. In the case of other OVD, a biopsy should be obtained at some point, whether at first evaluation or on follow-up.

Herpetic Lesions

The herpes family of viruses includes 8 members known to cause disease in humans. Herpes simplex virus type 1 (HSV1) is the causative agent in the vast majority of oral herpetic infections, as opposed to herpes simplex virus type 2 (HSV2), which is found mostly in genital infections.[26] However, either virus may be found in either location. Oral herpetic lesions are either primary (initial) or recurrent. Most people acquire HSV early in life through contact with mucous secretions (nasal, salivary) from someone who carries the virus. Carriers of the virus need not be symptomatic but may periodically shed the virus when it reactivates. These people are termed asymptomatic shedders. By age 70, 65% of the US population is seropositive for HSV.[27]

The individual who acquires HSV usually does not present with signs or symptoms. Forty-five minutes after exposure, 90% of viral particles have attached to a host cell.[28] However, in other individuals, the initial infection is quite prominent as well as painful and is called primary herpetic gingivostomatitis (PHG). PHG presents with multiple vesicles throughout the oral cavity that subsequently break down into ulcers. The clinical picture is accompanied by low-grade fever, malaise, oral pain, and lymphadenopathy.[29] The pain can be extensive, and talking and eating become difficult. PHG occurs in children, young adults, or the immunocompromised. Symptomatic treatment can include acetaminophen for the management of pain and fever. Topical local anesthetics such as 2% viscous lidocaine alone or mixed with diphenhydramine (ie, magic mouthwash) brings temporary relief.[26] Initiation of a systemic antiviral within the first 48 hours is recommended.[26,29,30] Acyclovir 200 mg, 5 times a day for 10 days, and valacyclovir 1000 mg twice a day for 10 days are useful options. Viral culture is confirmatory, but the result takes time.[29] The clinical picture of PHG is pathognomonic enough so as not to delay antiviral therapy.

In the case of oral herpes, HSV1 remains dormant in the trigeminal ganglia of infected individuals. HSV can be reactivated by several causes, such as a recent illness, excessive sun exposure, or a recent life stressor.[28] The recurrent forms of oral herpes present either as recurrent intraoral herpes (RIH) or as recurrent herpes labialis (RHL). The RIH form is found less commonly.[26] RIH presents on keratinized, attached oral mucosa as a cluster of several small vesicles in close proximity to one another. Thus, RIH would present on the buccal gingiva or the hard palate. The vesicles may breakdown and coalesce into a solitary ulcer. Clinically, they are similar in appearance to RAS, but RAS occurs on moveable mucosa instead of attached mucosa. RIH resolves without treatment within 2 weeks. Patients may be unaware of the presence of RIH because prodromal symptoms are usually not present.[26]

On the other hand, RHL does present with prodromal symptoms, and its appearance on the outer portion of the upper or lower lip can be a source of great embarrassment to the patient (**Fig. 7**). Prodromal symptoms that precede the development of the

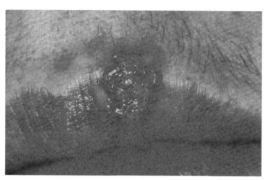

Fig. 7. RHL of the upper lip. RHL, when it recurs, usually erupts in the same area each time. In the first 5 days, the lesion is highly infectious. (*Courtesy of* Istvan A. Hargitai, DDS, MS, Bethesda, MD.)

RHL lesion include burning, itching, or tingling. RHL is found to occur in 20% to 40% of the general population.[27] In lay terms, RHL is called a "cold sore" or a "fever blister." The lesion manifests circa the mucocutaneous junction of the lip.

After viral reactivation via the previously mentioned causes, in 24 to 48 hours, vesicles appear on the lip and they coalesce into a single lesion. Within another 24 to 48 hours, the vesicles break down into an ulcer.[27] With the loss of the surface epithelium, nerve endings are more readily exposed and the lesion becomes painful. Stretching the lesion by smiling or eating can cause the ulcer to tear and bleeding may ensue. The clotting ulcer has a crusty appearance. The entire course of RHL resolves inside 2 weeks as the epithelium around the ulcer regenerates.

Because RHL is painful and the lesion is unsightly, patients often present for treatment. Within the first 4 to 5 days, the RHL lesion is teeming with virus. Patients must be instructed to avoid touching the lesion and then touching their eyes because they may self-inoculate. Patients must be told that in the first few days they are contagious and should avoid sharing utensils, cups, or letting others come in contact with the lesion.[23] RHL can be managed by topical or systemic antiviral medications. The topical antiviral creams are applied every 2 hours (during awake hours) at the first sign of the prodrome or the appearance of the vesicles and then continue for 4 to 5 days. After day 5, the lesion is usually no longer infectious. After applying the cream, the patient should wash their hands. Available antiviral creams include prescription acyclovir 5%, penciclovir 1%, and OTC docosanol 1%.[26,27,31] Although topicals may only shorten the duration of the lesion by a day, they do help reduce the severity of pain and appearance of the lesion.

Systemic antivirals are another option. They too must be implemented within 24 to 48 hours to be beneficial. Beyond 72 hours, they will not be helpful. The readily available options include acyclovir, valacyclovir, and famciclovir.[27,31] Acyclovir 400 mg at 3 times a day dosing for 5 days is the less expensive, older option. Valacyclovir is the prodrug of acyclovir and has 3 to 5 times the bioavailability of acyclovir.[27] Thus, a 1 day course of 1000 mg of valacyclovir given twice within the first day of the prodrome or vesicle appearance, can shorten the duration and decrease the severity of the RHL outbreak.[27] If there are greater than 6 RHL episodes per year, the clinician may consider placing the patient on suppressive, prophylactic therapy with a twice daily 500-mg dose of valacyclovir year round.[27] If sunlight is a known inducer of RHL outbreaks, the patient is instructed to apply daily lip balm with at least a 15 SPF (sun protection factor).

SUMMARY

Identification of OVD lesions and their subsequent treatment reduce pain and morbidity. Oral health care providers are familiar with the appearance of oral structures and architecture and are in an excellent position to identify or help identify oral lesions. Reducing oral pain and morbidity by managing these conditions is a great practice builder and establishes good patient rapport with dental, oral medicine, orofacial pain, or oral surgery practices.

REFERENCES

1. McCartan BE, Healy CM. The reported prevalence of oral lichen planus: a review and critique. J Oral Pathol Med 2008;37(8):447–53.
2. Lauritano D, Arrica M, Lucchese A, et al. Oral lichen planus clinical characteristics in Italian patients: a retrospective analysis. Head Face Med 2016;12:18.
3. Budimir V, Richter I, Andabak-Rogulj A, et al. Oral lichen planus - retrospective study of 563 Croatian patients. Med Oral Patol Oral Cir Bucal 2014;19(3): e255–60.
4. Chainani-Wu N, Silverman S Jr, Lozada-Nur F, et al. Oral lichen planus: patient profile, disease progression and treatment responses. J Am Dent Assoc 2001; 132(7):901–9.
5. Varghese SS, George GB, Sarojini SB, et al. Epidemiology of oral lichen planus in a cohort of south indian population: a retrospective study. J Cancer Prev 2016; 21(1):55–9.
6. Silverman S Jr, Bahl S. Oral lichen planus update: clinical characteristics, treatment responses, and malignant transformation. Am J Dent 1997;10(6):259–63.
7. Parashar P. Oral lichen planus. Otolaryngol Clin North Am 2011;44(1):89–107, vi.
8. Silverman S Jr, Gorsky M, Lozada-Nur F. A prospective follow-up study of 570 patients with oral lichen planus: persistence, remission, and malignant association. Oral Surg Oral Med Oral Pathol 1985;60(1):30–4.
9. Al-Hashimi I, Schifter M, Lockhart PB, et al. Oral lichen planus and oral lichenoid lesions: diagnostic and therapeutic considerations. Oral Surg Oral Med Oral Pathol Oral Radiol Endod 2007;103(Suppl):S25, e1–12.
10. Said S, Golitz L. Vesiculobullous eruptions of the oral cavity. Otolaryngol Clin North Am 2011;44(1):133–60, vi.
11. Kaplan I, Hodak E, Ackerman L, et al. Neoplasms associated with paraneoplastic pemphigus: a review with emphasis on non-hematologic malignancy and oral mucosal manifestations. Oral Oncol 2004;40(6):553–62.
12. McMillan R, Taylor J, Shephard M, et al. World workshop on oral medicine VI: a systematic review of the treatment of mucocutaneous pemphigus vulgaris. Oral Surg Oral Med Oral Pathol Oral Radiol 2015;120(2):132–42.e61.
13. Patel S, Kumar S, Laudenbach JM, et al. Mucocutaneous diseases: oral lichen planus, mucous membrane pemphigoid and pemphigus vulgaris. J Calif Dent Assoc 2016;44(9):561–70.
14. Gregoriou S, Efthymiou O, Stefanaki C, et al. Management of pemphigus vulgaris: challenges and solutions. Clin Cosmet Investig Dermatol 2015;8:521–7.
15. Broussard KC, Leung TG, Moradi A, et al. Autoimmune bullous diseases with skin and eye involvement: cicatricial pemphigoid, pemphigus vulgaris, and pemphigus paraneoplastica. Clin Dermatol 2016;34(2):205–13.
16. Terezhalmy GT, Bergfeld WF. Cicatricial pemphigoid (benign mucous membrane pemphigoid). Quintessence Int 1998;29(7):429–37.

17. Taylor J, McMillan R, Shephard M, et al. World workshop on oral medicine VI: a systematic review of the treatment of mucous membrane pemphigoid. Oral Surg Oral Med Oral Pathol Oral Radiol 2015;120(2):161–71.e20.
18. Haefliger S, Horn MP, Suter VG, et al. Rituximab for the treatment of isolated refractory desquamative gingivitis due to mucous membrane pemphigoid. JAMA Dermatol 2016;152(12):1396–8.
19. Yang MS, Lee JY, Kim J, et al. Incidence of Stevens-Johnson syndrome and toxic epidermal necrolysis: a nationwide population-based study using national health insurance database in Korea. PLoS One 2016;11(11):e0165933.
20. Celentano A, Tovaru S, Yap T, et al. Oral erythema multiforme: trends and clinical findings of a large retrospective European case series. Oral Surg Oral Med Oral Pathol Oral Radiol 2015;120(6):707–16.
21. Lozada-Nur F, Gorsky M, Silverman S Jr. Oral erythema multiforme: clinical observations and treatment of 95 patients. Oral Surg Oral Med Oral Pathol 1989;67(1): 36–40.
22. Lozada-Nur F, Cram D, Gorsky M. Clinical response to levamisole in thirty-nine patients with erythema multiforme. An open prospective study. Oral Surg Oral Med Oral Pathol 1992;74(3):294–8.
23. Silverman S Jr. Mucosal lesions in older adults. J Am Dent Assoc 2007; 138(Suppl):41S–6S.
24. Chattopadhyay A, Shetty KV. Recurrent aphthous stomatitis. Otolaryngol Clin North Am 2011;44(1):79–88, v.
25. Rodu B, Russell CM. Performance of a hydroxypropyl cellulose film former in normal and ulcerated oral mucosa. Oral Surg Oral Med Oral Pathol 1988;65(6): 699–703.
26. Stoopler ET, Balasubramaniam R. Topical and systemic therapies for oral and perioral herpes simplex virus infections. J Calif Dent Assoc 2013;41(4):259–62.
27. Woo SB, Challacombe SJ. Management of recurrent oral herpes simplex infections. Oral Surg Oral Med Oral Pathol Oral Radiol Endod 2007;103(Suppl):S12, e1–18.
28. Hicks ML, Terezhalmy GT. Herpesvirus hominis type 1: a summary of structure, composition, growth cycle, and cytopathogenic effects. Oral Surg Oral Med Oral Pathol 1979;48(4):311–8.
29. Chauvin PJ, Ajar AH. Acute herpetic gingivostomatitis in adults: a review of 13 cases, including diagnosis and management. J Can Dent Assoc 2002;68(4): 247–51.
30. Faden H. Management of primary herpetic gingivostomatitis in young children. Pediatr Emerg Care 2006;22(4):268–9.
31. Leung AKC, Barankin B. Herpes labialis: an update. Recent Pat Inflamm Allergy Drug Discov 2017;11(2):107–13.

Primary Headaches

Robert W. Mier, DDS, MS*, Shuchi Dhadwal, BDS, DMD

KEYWORDS

- Primary headache • Migraine • Tension-type headache
- Trigeminal autonomic cephalalgias • Cluster headache

KEY POINTS

- Primary headaches are defined by having the absence of an underlying pathologic process, disease, or traumatic injury that occurs in temporal relationship to the onset of pain.
- The primary headaches include migraine, tension-type headache, and the trigeminal autonomic cephalalgias (cluster headache, paroxysmal hemicranias, hemicrania continua, and short-lasting unilateral neuralgiform headaches with conjunctival injection and tearing/short-lasting unilateral neuralgiform headaches with cranial autonomic features syndrome).
- Advancements in understanding the pathophysiology have helped in more accurate diagnosis and efficacious treatments of these painful entities.
- New treatments have become available in recent years to help in treating these disorders using neuromodulation and newer classes of medications, including monoclonal antibodies, calcitonin gene-related peptide receptor antagonists, nontriptan serotonin receptor antagonists, and advances in triptan delivery.

INTRODUCTION

The primary headaches are disorders that exist with no apparent underlying cause with recurrent or persistent head pain, contrasted with the secondary headaches that exist in relation to discrete inciting factors. The exact mechanisms of these disorders have not been completely elucidated, but research continues to reveal more about the underlying pathophysiology and resultant treatment options. The primary headaches, according to the most recent iteration of the International Classification of Headache Disorders, Third Edition (ICHD-3), Beta Version,[1] consist of migraine, tension-type headache (TTH), the trigeminal autonomic cephalalgias (TACs), and various other primary headache disorders.

Headache, particularly in the chronic form, is a significant public health issue. TTH was the third most prevalent concern, with migraine reported to be the sixth most

Disclosure: The authors have nothing to disclose.
Tufts University School of Dental Medicine, 1 Kneeland Street, Suite 601, Boston, MA 02111, USA
* Corresponding author. 6730 South Harvard Drive, Franklin, WI 53132.
E-mail addresses: rwmier@gmail.com; bobmier@mac.com

prevalent concern in the 2016 Global Burden of Disease Study. Migraine was second only to lower back pain in the category Years Lived with Disability.[2]

The primary headaches share many common symptoms with an overlapping pathophysiology and treatment response. For diagnostic purposes, the ICHD divides primary headaches into discrete entities that use location, intensity, duration, accompaniments, and effective treatments to differentiate them.

The importance to dentistry lies in the fact that many patients who present with complaints of pain in the orofacial region may have a primary headache disorder. Thus it becomes incumbent on the dental profession to be knowledgeable of, and vigilant for, these disorders.

MIGRAINE

Migraine is a debilitating chronic neurologic disorder typically with an episodic presentation and significant comorbidities (**Boxes 1** and **2**). It can present in a chronic and a refractory form as well, both of which prove recalcitrant to conventional treatment and cause significant disability. The understanding of the pathophysiology has continued to evolve and now focuses on a centralized phenomenon that involves an altered sensory processing and excitability of the brain, originating in multiple brain areas and expressed predominantly in the trigeminovascular system. An in-depth discussion of the specifics of this complex issue is beyond the scope of this article but can be found in other publications.[3–7] The attacks are defined by unilateral head pain, throbbing in nature, and sensitivity to sensory input of sound, light, and movement. The pain can be from moderate to severe; it is the most disabling neurologic disorder and the sixth most disabling globally.[2,8]

Migraine exists with a 12% global prevalence (18% women, 6% men) and an incidence of 18.2 per 1000 in women aged 20 to 24 years and 6.2 per 1000 in men aged 15 to 19 years.[9,10] There is a 2.8:1 female to male ratio. This ratio diminishes at postmenopausal ages, and before puberty it favors men slightly. The median onset age is approximately the same for men and women at 24 to 25 years old.[11] It is accepted that migraine is a strongly heritable condition that is demonstrable as clusters within family groups; this is revealed to be a multifactorial genetic model, and this inherited susceptibility interacts with environmental factors to express the disorder.[12] Migraine with aura (MWA) and migraine without aura are distinct in their genetic heritability, and approximately one-third of patients experience MWA. It occurs more frequently in white people, and, in patients without a family history, prevalence increased with a decline in income.

The comorbid presence of other conditions is meaningful in migraine, including cardiovascular disease, epilepsy, asthma, sleep apnea, lupus, pain disorders, and

Box 1 Migraine	
Characteristics	Typically unilateral
	Pulsating
	Moderate/Severe pain level
	Aggravated by movement
	Individual often withdraws to quiet/dark setting
Accompaniments	Nausea and/or vomiting
	Photophobia and Phonophobia (at least one of the above)
Duration	4–72 h
Frequency	Episodic or chronic (>15 d)

Box 2
Migraine with aura

Characteristics	At least one reversible symptom that is visual, sensory, speech/language, motor, brainstem, or retinal
Accompaniments	Symptoms spread over minutes, and multiple ones can occur in succession
Duration	5–60 min with complete reversal of aura symptoms
Frequency	Headache phase follows the aura within 60 min, but can accompany it as well

Data from Headache Classification Committee of the International Headache Society (IHS). The international classification of headache disorders, 3rd edition (beta version). Cephalalgia 2013;33(9):629–808.

---

restless legs syndrome.[11] The vascular issues are significant and a thorough discussion is beyond the scope of this article but can be readily found in the literature. In addition, there is a significant comorbidity with depression and anxiety, with migraine symptoms most aggravated by anxiety.[13–15]

The presence of environmental triggers is a common issue and may include stress, lack of sleep or too much sleep, hunger, odors, bright lights, alcohol use, menses, foods, caffeine, and weather.[16,17] However, in some instances these stimuli are also symptoms of an attack already in progress. These issues apply to individuals with a genetic susceptibility to initiate the migraine phenomenon, which entails 4 main aspects, described as the prodrome (premonitory symptoms), the aura (if present), the headache phase, and the postdrome.

Prodrome

- Changes in mood (irritability)
- Fatigue
- Food cravings
- Yawning
- Neck stiffness
- Phonophobia
- Difficulty with concentration

Aura (Occurring in One-Third of Patients)

- Consists of transient neurologic deficits, described in **Box 2**
- Visual (positive [fortification, spectra], negative [scotoma], or both) disturbance occurs in 90% of patients who have aura
- Sensory, motor, speech, brain stem, and retinal disturbances
- Caused by a cortical spreading depression, not necessary to trigger the headache phase

Headache

- Described in **Boxes 1** and **2**
- Unilateral, throbbing, moderate-severe intensity, 4 to 72 hours duration
- Accompanied by nausea, photophobia and phonophobia, or both
- Aggravated by physical activity
- Often (>50%) accompanied by autonomic signs (especially tearing) and bilateral, which discriminates from TACs
- If present greater than 15 days a month is defined as chronic migraine

Postdrome

- Similar to the prodromal symptoms
- Fatigue, feeling washed out
- Difficulty concentrating
- Neck stiffness
- Often attributed to abortive medication effects by the patient
- Some symptoms may extend from the prodrome through to the postdrome stage

Neuroimaging studies such as structural brain imaging, MRI, functional MRI, and PET have been used to study discrete structural, blood flow, metabolic, sensory, and resting-state differences between migraineurs and controls. This approach has produced reliable discriminators in visual, somatosensory, auditory, and nociceptive aspects for patients with migraine. These differences remain consistent even during interictal periods. Taken with the findings in bench, laboratory, and clinical situations, the understanding of migraine as a primary brain dysfunction has developed.[3]

The differential diagnosis of migraine must entail ruling out secondary causes first. This diagnosis is best evaluated with a mnemonic device from Dr. David Dodick[18] termed SSNOOPP. This mnemonic delineates in a simplistic manner the red flags to be aware of when evaluating a patient with headache:

- Systemic symptoms (fever, weight loss)
- Secondary risk factors from underlying disease (human immunodeficiency virus, cancer, autoimmune disorder)
- Neurologic symptoms or abnormal signs (confusion, motor or sensory deficits, impaired alertness, abnormal focal examination)
- Onset: sudden, abrupt, or split-second onset; first or worst headache
- Older age onset: new and progressive headache, especially greater than 50 years old
- Pattern change: first headache or a change from existing headache pattern
- Previous headache history: change in frequency, severity, or clinical features

A positive indicator for headache from a secondary cause warrants a referral to a neurologist/headache specialist to prevent delay in diagnosis and treatment. Many of the secondary entities can mimic an episodic or chronic benign headache syndrome, including dental, jaw, and oral disorders. Although patients with these red flags may not necessarily have secondary headache disorders, further investigation is always the most prudent course of action. Once the issue of secondary headache is eliminated, the classification of a primary headache disorder can follow based on history and clinical examination.

Treatment of migraine involves both abortive and preventive strategies. The primary goal is to reduce pain and restore function/quality of life but additionally is to prevent the progression from episodic migraine (EM) to chronic migraine (CM) that occurs approximately 2.5%/y.[19] Treatment strategies should include patient education, lifestyle modifications, management of triggers, and acute/preventive pharmacology. Not every patient with EM needs preventive therapy, but all patients with CM do. The treatments are listed in **Table 1**, with the understanding that no single treatment is effective for all patients. Therapy needs to be tailored to the individual, and often an incremental approach to management is required because improvement is realized over time. Acute treatment should be tailored to the disability of the attack and preventive therapy to the activity of the disorder. Despite this approach, adherence to preventive medication is only 25% at 6 months and 14% at 1 year. In addition,

Table 1
Treatment options for migraine (level A evidence)

Headache Type	Migraine (Episodic)	Migraine (Chronic)
Nonpharmacologic treatment options	Explanation of headache mechanism, treatments available, and prognosis. Include discussion of MOH risks (>8 d/mo use of abortive agent). Use of headache diary Avoidance of known triggers (eg, alcohol, nitroglycerin, daytime napping, untreated apnea, stress) Cognitive behavior therapy, biofeedback, relaxation techniques, acupuncture	Same as episodic
First-line treatment Abortive	Triptans: oral, nasal, injectable, transdermal Best to limit use to 2–3 times/wk, use as early in headache phase as possible Sumatriptan: 25, 50, 100 mg oral; 10, 20 mg nasal; 6 SC Zolmitriptan: 2.5, 5 mg oral; 2.5, 5 mg nasal Rizatriptan: 10 mg oral Naratriptan: 2.5 mg oral Eletriptan: 20, 40 mg oral Almotriptan: 12.5 mg oral Frovatriptan: 2.5 mg oral (efficacious in menstrual migraine with proper protocol) NSAIDs: ASA, ibuprofen 200–800 mg, naproxen 500–1000 mg, diclofenac 50–100 mg, diclofenac potassium oral solution, paracetamol 1000 mg Dihydroergotamine tablets and nasal sprays	Not effective, increased risk of MOH
Preventive	Propranolol 40–240 mg Metoprolol 50–200 mg Timolol 10–30 mg Valproic acid 500–1800 mg Topiramate 25–100 mg *Petasites* (butterbur) 75 mg BID Amitriptyline 50–150 mg (level B, probably effective)	Onabotulinum toxin A Injection protocol
Benefit from neuromodulation/ type	Yes Hypothalamus GON unilateral and bilateral SPG High cervical spinal Vagal	May benefit in select patients

Abbreviations: ASA, acetylsalicylic acid; BID, twice a day; GON, greater occipital nerve; MOH, medication overuse headache; NSAIDs, nonsteroidal anti-inflammatory drugs; SC, subcutaneous; SPG, sphenopalatine ganglion.
Data from Refs.[19–28]

switching among medications is common and most patients do not remain on the initial triptan prescribed.[29]

New therapeutic approaches are being developed to improve both effectiveness in pain reduction and compliance in episodic, chronic, and refractory migraine.[3,20,30–32] The following are currently under investigation or in use:

- Monoclonal antibodies: targeting calcitonin gene-related peptide (CGRP) as a preventive agent, no liver toxicity, early results are encouraging, cost may be an issue, must be injected or infused. Monoclonal antibodies hold the most promise for success in refractory and chronic cases. In May 2018 the FDA approved Erenumab (Aimovig) as the first drug in this class for patient use with several more expected to be approved soon.
- CGRP antagonists (gepants): oral delivery, but issues with liver toxicity.
- Nontriptan serotonin receptor antagonists: oral delivery, no vasoconstriction so a significant adverse effect of the triptans is avoided, and an agonist of the 5-hydroxytryptamine 1F receptor.
- Alternative delivery systems for existing medications: intranasal delivery of sumatriptan, autoinjector 3 mg sumatriptan, transdermal iontophoretic delivery of sumatriptan, oral inhalation of dihydroergotamine for benefit in the late headache phase, and inhaled and microneedle patch for zolmitriptan.
- Noninvasive neuromodulation: transcranial magnetic stimulation, transcranial direct current stimulation, pericranial peripheral nerve stimulation, and vagal nerve stimulation.
- Implantable neuromodulation: occipital nerve stimulation, sphenopalatine ganglion stimulation, and high cervical spinal cord stimulation.

TENSION-TYPE HEADACHE

TTH is a primary headache characterized as mild to moderate head pain that is not associated with nausea and vomiting, but photophobia or phonophobia may be present.[1] Pain is pressing or tightening in quality and located bilaterally in the temple and occipital areas (**Box 3**).

The ICHD classifies TTH as infrequent episodic, frequent episodic, chronic, and probable. Chronic TTH (CTTH) is characterized by more than 15 d/mo of headache.

TTH is the most common primary headache disorder, and a cross-sectional study suggested that TTH affects women slightly more than men, with average onset age of 25 to 30 years and peak age of 39 years.[33] TTH has a global prevalence of 38% and lifetime prevalence of 46%.[34] CTTH affects 0.5% to 4.8% of the population worldwide.

Although the pathophysiology of TTH is unclear, peripheral mechanisms of pericranial tenderness, a generalized pressure pain hypersensitivity, and muscle tightness play a vital role in the development of TTH.[35] Central mechanisms expressed as central sensitivity likely play an important role in CTTH. Genetic studies suggest familial aggregation of TTH and an inherited susceptibility as well. Psychological factors play a crucial role in many patients, particularly in patients with CTTH.[36]

Box 3 Tension-type headache	
Characteristics	Bilateral, pressing quality (tight headband), mild/moderate pain, not aggravated by movement
Accompaniments	No nausea/vomiting, either photophobia or phonophobia
Duration	30 min to 7 d
Frequency	Episodic or chronic

Data from Headache Classification Committee of the International Headache Society (IHS). The international classification of headache disorders, 3rd edition (beta version). Cephalalgia 2013;33(9):629–808.

Comprehensive history taking is the key because it can help clinicians differentiate between TTH and other primary and secondary headaches.[37]

Clinicians often have difficulty distinguishing between TTH and migraine without aura. Therefore, a detailed history and examination, along with a pain diary to study the pattern of the headaches, can be helpful in gathering the information and making the correct diagnosis. Manual palpation of masticatory and cervical muscles should be performed, and muscular trigger points with pericranial tenderness may be present.[38]

Pharmacologic Treatment

Nonsteroidal antiinflammatory drugs are the first choice of therapy for episodic TTH and combination analgesics are often the second choice (**Table 2**). A low-dose tricyclic antidepressant, such as amitriptyline 10 to 50 mg, is the first-line treatment of CTTH.[39]

Nonpharmacologic Treatment

Cognitive behavior therapy, biofeedback, and mindfulness are helpful in decreasing the pain intensity and headache-related disability in patients with CTTH.[40] There is sufficient evidence to support that acupuncture is an effective short-term treatment of frequent episodic and chronic TTH.[41]

A study by Epsi-Lopez and colleagues[42] investigated the effects of manual therapy techniques in patients with TTH and CTTH. At 4 weeks, patients in the treatment group reported improvement in quality of life, improved function, and decreased pain intensity.

There is little evidence that occlusal stabilization splints or irreversible dental treatments are effective in reducing the frequency of CTTH despite anecdotal reports of benefit, thus further long-term studies are needed to establish the role of appliance therapy for treatment of CTTH.[43,44]

Table 2
Treatment options for tension-type headache

Substance	Dose (mg)	Level of Recommendation	Comment
Ibuprofen	200–800	A	Gastrointestinal side effects, risk of bleeding
Ketoprofen	25	A	Side effects as for ibuprofen
Aspirin	500–1000	A	Side effects as for ibuprofen
Naproxen	375–550	A	Side effects as for ibuprofen
Diclofenac	12.5–100	A	Side effects as for ibuprofen, only doses of 12.5–25 mg tested in TTH
Paracetamol caffeine combination	1000 (oral) 65–200	A B	Less risk of gastrointestinal side effects compared with NSAIDs (discussed later)[a]

The level of recommendation considers side effects and consistency of the studies. There is sparse evidence for optimal doses. The most effective dose of a drug well tolerated by a patient should be chosen.

[a] Combination with caffeine 65 to 200 mg increases the efficacy of ibuprofen[43] and paracetamol.[31,42] but possibly also the risk for developing use headache.[46,53] Level of recommendation of combination drugs containing caffeine is therefore B.

From Bendtsen L, Evers S, Linde M, et al. EFNS guideline on the treatment of tension-type headache - report of an EFNS task force. Eur J Neurol 2010;17(11):1318–25; with permission.

TRIGEMINAL AUTONOMIC CEPHALALGIAS

The TACs (**Table 3**) are a group of disorders characterized by a lateralized symptom of prominent headache in the orbital, supraorbital, and temporal regions (but may include other sites within the trigeminal nerve distribution) and accompanied by ipsilateral cranial autonomic features of conjunctival injection, periorbital edema, facial flushing, otic fullness, lacrimation, and rhinorrhea.[1] The TACs include cluster headache (CH), paroxysmal hemicrania (PH), short-lasting unilateral neuralgiform headaches with conjunctival injection and tearing (SUNCT), short-lasting unilateral neuralgiform headaches with cranial autonomic features (SUNA), and hemicrania continua (HC). These disorders are distinguished by their attack duration, frequency, and response to treatment.

An important distinction from other primary headaches is the unilaterality of photophobia or phonophobia ipsilateral to the pain, and it may be up to 10 times as common in TACs than in migraine.[45] Another hallmark of the TACs is the presence of agitation in patients who experience them, likely caused by activation of the posterior hypothalamus.[46–50]

The addition of neuroimaging studies has allowed clinicians to understand the importance of the hypothalamus in the pathophysiology of TACs. It is thought that this area of the brain regulates duration of attacks, and differing responses would help explain the nuances between the presentations of the TACs. The issue is now understood to be more complex and involves the entire pain matrix (ie, angular cingulate cortex, contralateral posterior thalamus, ipsilateral basal ganglia, bilateral insulae, periaqueductal gray, rostral ventral medulla, and the cerebellar hemisphere), which allows a more centralized and permissive pain state.[51–55]

Although TACs are considered primary headache syndromes, a percentage of these presentations can be from secondary causes. Pituitary gland, posterior fossa, maxillary sinus, orbital and upper cervical disorders of differing natures can present with TAC-like symptoms.[56,57]

Cluster Headache

CH (see **Table 3; Box 4**), the epitome of the TACs, presents as dominantly retro-orbital pain (70%) described as a boring, stabbing, burning, or squeezing. The pain is among the worst in human experience and leaves the patients restless and agitated. The core feature that gives CH its name is the circadian periodicity relative to active/inactive episodes over time. There is a predilection for the first rapid eye movement cycle in sleep, and a comorbidity with obstructive sleep apnea.[58] Most active episodic cluster periods last 2 to 12 weeks. The remission periods may last between 6 and 24 months. There is a prevalence of 0.1% to 0.4% and significant disability because of the severity of pain.[59–61] The typical age of onset is 20 to 40 years.[62]

The pathophysiology of cluster headache involves a peripheral trigeminal component that is validated by levels of CGRP,[63,64] the benefit of triptans in resolving CH attacks, and the symptoms evident in secondary cases. However, the presence of pain outside the trigeminal distribution, lack of benefit from trigeminal surgical lesioning, and continued triptan benefit after lesioning[65] reinforces the lack of a primary peripheral generator. A central component presents itself as a centralized permissive state via major effects on the hypothalamus and descending pain inhibitory network.

Treatment of CH is mandatory, and involves abortive and preventive strategies (**Table 4**).

The issue of medically refractory cases has been a concern in the treatment of CHs, and recently hypothalamic, greater occipital nerve, vagal nerve, high cervical spinal cord, and sphenopalatine ganglion stimulation have been used with significant

Table 3
Comparison of the trigeminal autonomic cephalalgias

Headache Type	Cluster Headache	Paroxysmal Hemicrania	SUNCT/SUNA	Hemicrania Continua
Sex	3 M to 1 F	M = F	1.5 M to 1 F	1 M to 1.6 F
Pain				
Quality	Sharp/stab/throb	Sharp/stab/throb	Sharp/stab/throb	Throbbing/sharp/constant
Severity	Very severe	Very severe	Severe	Moderate to severe
Distribution	V1>C2>V2>V3	V1>C2>V2>V3	V1>C2>V2>V3	V1>C2>V2>V3
Attacks				
Frequency/d	1–8	11	100	Continuous with exacerbations
Duration (min)	15–180	2–30	1–10	
Triggering	Absent	Absent	Present	Absent
Agitation (%)	90	80	65	69
Episodic vs chronic	90:10	35:65	10:90	15:85
Periodicity	Present	Absent	Absent	Absent
Treatment Effects				
Oxygen (%)	70	No effect	No effect	No effect
Sumatriptan (%)	90	20	<10	No effect
Indomethacin (%)	No effect	100	No effect	100
Migraine Features				
Nausea (%)	50	40	25	53
Photophobia (%)	65	65	25	79
Phonophobia (%)	—	—	—	—

Abbreviations: C, cervical; F, female; M, male; V, trigeminal.
From Eller M, Goadsby PJ. Trigeminal autonomic cephalalgias. Oral Dis 2016;222(1); with permission.

Box 4	
Cluster headache	
Characteristics	Severe/very severe pain; unilateral with temporal or periorbital location
Accompaniments	Ipsilateral autonomic signs/symptoms with at least one of tearing/conjunctival injection, nasal congestion/runny nose, eyelid swelling, facial sweating/flushing, ear fullness, and miosis/ptosis. Individual demonstrates an agitated demeanor
Duration	15–180 min
Frequency	Varies between 1–8/d within periods of activity, which may be followed by significant periods of inactivity in an often circadian rhythmicity

Data from Headache Classification Committee of the International Headache Society (IHS). The international classification of headache disorders, 3rd edition (beta version). Cephalalgia 2013;33(9):629–808.

success in approximately 66% of patients.[71–74] The hypothalamic stimulation is not effective acutely but requires weeks to months before benefit may be realized. Radiofrequency ablation via thermocoagulation has been a mainstay for surgical treatment of cluster but, with improving benefits from the use of stimulators, this technique-sensitive destructive approach should find less use.

SHORT-LASTING UNILATERAL NEURALGIFORM HEADACHE WITH CONJUNCTIVAL INJECTION AND TEARING/CRANIAL AUTONOMIC SYMPTOMS)

The syndromes of SUNCT/SUNA are composed of brief attacks of moderate/severe unilateral head and/or facial pain associated with cranial autonomic symptoms (**Box 5**). SUNA is differentiated by the presence of 1 or neither of lacrimation or conjunctival injection. There is typically an absence of nausea, photophobia, and phonophobia.[75–77] Pain presents as orbital, supraorbital, or temporal, but may arise anywhere in the head and is described as burning, stabbing, or electric. There is typically a cutaneous trigger as with trigeminal neuralgia (TN), but it can be spontaneous as well. However, unlike TN, there is no refractory period. There is also no tendency toward nocturnal attacks.[55,62,66–68]

SUNCT/SUNA have a prevalence of 6.6 to 109 per 100,000,[59,78] an incidence of 1.2 per 100,000,[78] and age at onset from 35 to 65 years(mean, 48 years).[79] SUNA may have a slight female dominance.

The pathophysiology of SUNCT/SUNA is again associated with the hypothalamus and the trigeminal system, as discussed with cluster. However, owing to the clinical similarities with TN, there is the potential involvement of vascular compression of the trigeminal nerve.[55,80] Secondary causes may involve pituitary, posterior fossa, and trigeminal nerve disorders.

Treatment of SUNCT/SUNA (see **Table 4**) has proved resistant to medical treatment in many instances, and the options in surgical management have evolved from destructive lesioning of the trigeminal nerve to now include microvascular decompression procedures as well as vagal, greater occipital nerve, sphenopalatine ganglion, and hypothalamic stimulation with benefit and much fewer adverse effects in approximately two-thirds of patients.[55,74,79,81–93]

PAROXYSMAL HEMICRANIA/HEMICRANIA CONTINUA

These two variants of the TAC family are grouped together and defined by their absolute response to indomethacin, but they do present differently clinically.

Table 4
Treatment options for the trigeminal autonomic cephalgias

Headache Type	CH	Paroxysmal Hemicrania	SUNCT/SUNA	Hemicrania Continua
Nonpharmacologic treatment options	Explanation of headache mechanism, treatments available, and prognosis. Include discussion of MOH risks Avoidance of known triggers (eg, alcohol, nitroglycerin, daytime napping, untreated apnea, stress)	Explanation to patient as with CH	Explanation to patient as with CH Avoidance of cutaneous triggers if present	Explanation to patient as with cluster headache
First-line treatment Abortive (% response)	12–15 L/min O$_2$ (70%) Sumatriptan SC 6 mg (90%)	Indomethacin (100%) 25 mg/d titrating to 150 mg/d TID	None because of short pain duration	Indomethacin (100%) 25 mg/d titrating to 150 mg/d TID
Preventive	Verapamil 80 mg TID to start, titrating by 80 mg every 3–7 d (caution for ECG because of risk of heart block)		Lamotrigine 25 mg BID to start and titrating in 25-mg increments every 7–14 d	
Alternative treatment Abortive	Zolmitriptan 10 mg Dihydroergotamine IM or nasal spray Intranasal lidocaine GON blocks	GON blocks	None	GON blocks
Preventive	Corticosteroid: prednisone 80 mg with 10-d/2-mg taper (for transitional use) Lithium Valproic acid Topiramate Melatonin	Topiramate Melatonin Alternative NSAID	Topiramate Gabapentinoids Zonisamide IV lidocaine Carbamazepine Oxcarbazepine	Topiramate Melatonin Alternative NSAID
Benefit from neuromodulation/type	Yes Hypothalamus GON unilateral and bilateral SPG High cervical spinal Vagal	Yes Hypothalamus GON unilateral SPG	Yes Hypothalamus GON bilateral SPG Vagal Surgical: microvascular decompression of trigeminal nerve root	Yes Hypothalamus GON unilateral SPG

Abbreviations: ECG, electrocardiogram; IM, intramuscular; IV, intravenous; TID, 3 times a day.
Data from Refs.[31,55,62,66–70]

Box 5 SUNCT/SUNA	
Characteristics	Moderate/severe unilateral pain; trigeminal distribution but typically temporal and periorbital, and often a trigger zone similar to trigeminal neuralgia
Accompaniments	Ipsilateral autonomic signs/symptoms with at least one of tearing/conjunctival injection, nasal congestion/runny nose, eyelid swelling, facial sweating/flushing, ear fullness, and miosis/ptosis
Duration	1–600 s
Frequency	At least once/day

Data from Headache Classification Committee of the International Headache Society (IHS). The international classification of headache disorders, 3rd edition (beta version). Cephalalgia 2013;33(9):629–808.

PH is a rare condition (0.5 per 1000 or less) marked by short attacks of unilateral orbital, temporal, and above or behind the ear pain (**Box 6**). The attacks are spontaneous, but approximately 10% may arise from mechanical neck triggers. The pain is described as boring, clawlike, or pulsatile. Attacks are side-locked but may alternate sides between attacks. There are prominent cranial autonomic symptoms as with the other TACs, and dominated by tearing.[62]

HC is described as a continuous unilateral and side-locked headache in the temporal or periorbital regions that varies in intensity without complete resolution[94] (**Box 7**). There may be aura associated with attacks as well.[95] To further differentiate from PH, the background pain of HC is greater than the interparoxysmal pain of the other TACs, and the exacerbations of pain last longer.[68]

The pathophysiology is assumed to be consistent with hypothalamic and trigeminal dysfunction, with a diminished descending pain inhibitory system and a resultant central permissive state. It is of interest to note that these two entities, and to some degree the other TACs as well, are often misdiagnosed with dental or temporomandibular joint pain.[96–99]

Treatment (see **Table 4**) is an absolute response to indomethacin starting at 25 mg/d and titrating up to 150 mg on a 3-times-a-day regimen. In addition, benefit has been shown with the use of greater occipital blocks and stimulation.[91,94,100–109]

Differential Diagnosis of Trigeminal Autonomic Cephalalgias and Dental Considerations

It is common for patients with TACs to consult dentists for diagnosis. CH is often misdiagnosed as migraine, TN, odontogenic pain, and sinus headache/infection. As

Box 6 Paroxysmal hemicrania	
Characteristics	Severe unilateral pain; temporal and periorbital in location. Sensitive to indomethacin
Accompaniments	Ipsilateral autonomic signs/symptoms with at least one of tearing/conjunctival injection, nasal congestion/runny nose, eyelid swelling, facial sweating/flushing, ear fullness, and miosis/ptosis
Duration	2–30 min
Frequency	Greater than 5/d

Data from Headache Classification Committee of the International Headache Society (IHS). The international classification of headache disorders, 3rd edition (beta version). Cephalalgia 2013;33(9):629–808.

Box 7	
Hemicrania continua	
Characteristics	Constant and side-locked moderate/severe head pain in a temporal and periorbital location. Sensitive to indomethacin
Accompaniments	Ipsilateral autonomic signs/symptoms with at least one of tearing/ conjunctival injection, nasal congestion/runny nose, eyelid swelling, facial sweating/flushing, ear fullness, and miosis/ptosis
Duration	Constant but can vary in intensity
Frequency	Constant and unrelenting

Data from Headache Classification Committee of the International Headache Society (IHS). The international classification of headache disorders, 3rd edition (beta version). Cephalalgia 2013;33(9):629–808.

mentioned previously, HC and PH are often misdiagnosed as odontogenic, temporomandibular pain, TN, or cervicogenic headache. SUNCT/SUNA are primarily misdiagnosed as TN owing to the significant overlap in symptoms, but they are misdiagnosed as odontogenic pain as well. The primary issue stems from nonheadache specialists being unaware of these less common presentations and the nuances involved in understanding the clues in history and presentation that help discern differences.[98]

OTHER PRIMARY HEADACHES

The ICHD-3 lists 10 other varieties of primary headache. The scope of the current article prohibits complete descriptions here, but the reader is referred to the ICHD and accompanying references. The ICHD-3 (beta) may be found at https://www.ichd-3.org/

REFERENCES

1. Headache Classification Committee of the International Headache Society (IHS). The international classification of headache disorders, 3rd edition (beta version). Cephalagia 2013;33:629–808.
2. Abajobir AA, Abate KH, Abbafati C, et al. Global, regional, and national incidence, prevalence, and years lived with disability for 328 diseases and injuries for 195 countries, 1990–2016: a systematic analysis for the Global Burden of Disease Study 2016. Lancet 2017;390(10100):1211–59.
3. Goadsby PJ, Holland PR, Martins-Oliveira M, et al. Pathophysiology of migraine: a disorder of sensory processing. Physiol Rev 2017;97(2):553–622.
4. Charles A. Advances in the basic and clinical science of migraine. Ann Neurol 2009;65(5):491–8.
5. Edvinsson L. Basic mechanisms of migraine and its acute treatment. Pharmacol Ther 2012;136:319–33.
6. Goadsby PJ. Migraine pathophysiology. Headache 2005;45(Suppl 1):S14–24.
7. Goadsby PJ. Pathophysiology of migraine. Neurol Clin 2009;27(2):335–60.
8. Global Burden of Disease Study 2013 Collaborators. Global, regional, and national incidence, prevalence, and years lived with disability for 301 acute and chronic diseases and injuries in 188 countries. Lancet 2015;386:743–800.
9. Lipton RB, Bigal ME, Diamond M, et al, AMPP Advisory Group. Migraine prevalence, disease burden, and the need for preventive therapy. Neurology 2007;68(5):343–9.

10. Stewart WF, Wood C, Reed ML, et al, AMPP Advisory Group. Cumulative lifetime migraine incidence in women and men. Cephalagia 2008;28(11):1170–8.
11. Robbins MS, Lipton RB. The epidemiology of primary headache disorders. Semin Neurol 2010;30(2):107–19.
12. Silberstein SD, Dodick DW. Migraine genetics: part II. Headache 2013;53(8):1218–29.
13. Zwart JA, Dyb G, Hagen K, et al. Depression and anxiety disorders associated with headache frequency. The Nord-Trondelag Health Study. Eur J Neurol 2003;10(2):147–52.
14. Jette N, Patten S, Williams J, et al. Comorbidity of migraine and psychiatric disorders–a national population-based study. Headache 2008;48(4):501–16.
15. Smitherman TA, Penzien DB, Maizels M. Anxiety disorders and migraine intractability and progression. Curr Pain Headache Rep 2008;12(3):224–9.
16. Andress-Rothrock D, King W, Rothrock J. An analysis of migraine triggers in a clinic-based population. Headache 2010;50(8):1366–70.
17. Kelman L. The triggers or precipitants of the acute migraine attack. Cephalalgia 2007;27(5):394–402.
18. Dodick DW. Clinical clues and clinical rules: primary versus secondary headache. Adv Stud Med 2003;3:S550–5.
19. Bigal ME, Serrano D, Buse D, et al. Acute migraine medications and evolution from episodic to chronic migraine: a longitudinal population-based study. Headache 2008;48:1157–68.
20. Lipton RB, Sillberstein SD. Episodic and chronic migraine headache: breaking down barriers to optimal treatment and prevention. Headache 2015;55:99–102.
21. Becker WJ. Acute migraine treatment in adults. Headache 2015;55(6):778–93.
22. Evers S, Afra J, Frese A, et al. EFNS guideline on the drug treatment of migraine–revised report of an EFNS task force. Eur J Neurol 2009;16(9):968–81.
23. Holland S, Silberstein SD, Freitag F, et al. Evidence-based guideline update: NSAIDs and other complementary treatments for episodic migraine prevention in adults. Neurology 2012;78:1346–53.
24. Loder E, Burch R, Rizzoli P. The 2012 AHS/AAN guidelines for prevention of episodic migraine: a summary and comparison with other recent clinical practice guidelines. Headache 2012;52(6):930–45.
25. Silberstein S, Holland S, Freitag F, et al. Evidence-based guideline update: pharmacologic treatment for episodic migraine prevention in adults. Neurology 2012;78:1337–45.
26. Bigal ME, Lipton RB. The differential diagnosis of chronic daily headaches: an algorithm-based approach. J Headache Pain 2007;8(5):263–72.
27. Aurora SK, Dodick DW, Turkel CC, et al. OnabotulinumtoxinA for treatment of chronic migraine: results from the double-blind, randomized, placebo-controlled phase of the PREEMPT 1 trial. Cephalalgia 2010;30(7):793–803.
28. Diener HC, Dodick DW, Aurora SK, et al. OnabotulinumtoxinA for treatment of chronic migraine: results from the double-blind, randomized, placebo-controlled phase of the PREEMPT 2 trial. Cephalalgia 2010;30(7):804–14.
29. Hepp Z, Dodick DW, Varon SF, et al. Persistence and switching patterns of oral migraine prophylactic medications among patients with chronic migraine: a retrospective claims analysis. Cephalalgia 2017;37(5):470–85.
30. Maasumi K. New treatments for headache. Neurol Sci 2017;38(Suppl 1):145–56.
31. Schuster NM, Rapoport AM. New strategies for the treatment and prevention of primary headache disorders. Nat Rev Neurol 2016;12(11):635–50.

32. Puledda F, Messina R, Goadsby PJ. An update on migraine: current understanding and future directions. J Neurol 2017;264(9):2031–9.
33. Lyngberg AC, Rasmussen BK, Jorgensen T, et al. Has the prevalence of migraine and tension-type headache changed over a 12-year period? A Danish population survey. Eur J Epidemiol 2005;20(3):243–9.
34. Stovner L, Hagen K, Jensen R, et al. The global burden of headache: a documentation of headache prevalence and disability worldwide. Cephalalgia 2007;27(3):193–210.
35. Ashina S, Bendtsen L, Ashina M. Pathophysiology of tension-type headache. Curr Pain Headache Rep 2005;9(6):415–22.
36. Yu S, Han X. Update of chronic tension-type headache. Curr Pain Headache Rep 2015;19(1):469.
37. Ravishankar K. The art of history-taking in a headache patient. Ann Indian Acad Neurol 2012;15(Suppl 1):S7–14.
38. Jensen RH. Tension-type headache – the normal and most prevalent headache. Headache 2018;58(2):339–45.
39. Bendtsen L, Evers S, Linde M, et al. EFNS guideline on the treatment of tension-type headache - report of an EFNS task force. Eur J Neurol 2010;17(11):1318–25.
40. Probyn K, Bowers H, Mistry D, et al. Non-pharmacological self-management for people living with migraine or tension-type headache: a systematic review including analysis of intervention components. BMJ Open 2017;7(8):e016670.
41. Linde K, Allais G, Brinkhaus B, et al. Acupuncture for the prevention of tension-type headache. Cochrane Database Syst Rev 2016;(4):CD007587.
42. Espi-Lopez GV, Rodriguez-Blanco C, Oliva-Pascual-Vaca A, et al. Do manual therapy techniques have a positive effect on quality of life in people with tension-type headache? A randomized controlled trial. Eur J Phys Rehabil Med 2016;52(4):447–56.
43. Kostrzewa-Janicka J, Mierzwinska-Nastalska E, Rolski D, et al. Occlusal stabilization splint therapy in orofacial pain and tension-type headache. Adv Exp Med Biol 2013;788:181–8.
44. Troeltzsch M, Messlinger K, Brodine B, et al. A comparison of conservative and invasive dental approaches in the treatment of tension-type headache. Quintessence Int 2014;45(9):795–802.
45. Irimia P, Cittadini E, Paemeleire K, et al. Unilateral photophobia or phonophobia in migraine compared with trigeminal autonomic cephalalgias. Cephalagia 2008;28(6):626–30.
46. Cohen AS. Short-lasting unilateral neuralgiform headache attacks with conjunctival injection and tearing. Cephalagia 2007;27:824–32.
47. Matharu MS, Cohen AS, McGonigle DJ, et al. Posterior hypothalamic and brainstem activation in hemicrania continua. Headache 2004;44:747–61.
48. Matharu MS, Cohen AS, Frackowiak RSJ, et al. Posterior hypothalamic activation in paroxysmal hemicrania. Ann Neurol 2006;59:535–45.
49. May A, Bahra A, Buchel C, Frackowiak RS, Goadsby PJ. Hypothalamic activation in cluster headache attacks. Lancet 1998;352:275–8.
50. May A, Bahra A, Buchel C, et al. Functional MRI in spontaneous attacks of SUNCT: short-lasting neuralgiform headache with conjunctival injection and tearing. Ann Neurol 1999;46:791–3.
51. Zukerman E, Peres MF, Kaup AO, et al. Chronic paroxysmal hemicrania-tic syndrome. Neurology 2000;54(7):1524–6.
52. Green M, Apfelbaum R. Cluster-tic syndrome headache. Headache 1978;18:112.

53. Solomon S, Apfelbaum RI, Guglielmo KM. The cluster-tic syndrome and its surgical therapy. Cephalagia 1985;5(2):83–9.
54. Wilbrink LA, Weller CM, Cheung C, et al. Cluster-tic syndrome: a cross-sectional study of cluster headache patients. Headache 2013;53:1334–40.
55. Benoliel R, Sharav Y, Haviv Y, et al. Tic, triggering, and tearing: from CTN to SU-NHA. Headache 2017;57(6):997–1009.
56. Favier I, van Vliet JA, Roon KI, et al. Trigeminal autonomic cephalgias due to structural lesions: a review of 31 cases. Arch Neurol 2007;64:25–31.
57. Levy M, Matharu Meeran K, Powell M, et al. The clinical characteristics of headache in patients with pituitary tumours. Brain 2005;128:1921–30.
58. Graff-Radford SB, Newman A. Obstructive sleep apnea and cluster headache. Headache 2004;44:607–10.
59. Sjaastad O, Bakketeig LS. Cluster headache prevalence. Vaga study of headache epidemiology. Cephalagia 2003;23(7):528–33.
60. Ekbom K, Svensson DA, Pedersen NL, et al. Lifetime prevalence and concordance risk of cluster headache in the Swedish twin population. Neurology 2006;67:798–803.
61. Torelli P, Beghi E, Manzoni GC. Cluster headache prevalence in the Italian general population. Neurology 2005;64:469–74.
62. Rozen TD. Trigeminal autonomic cephalalgias. Neurol Clin 2009;27(2):537–56.
63. Goadsby PJ, Edvinsson L. Human in vivo evidence for trigeminovascular activation in cluster headache. Neuropeptide changes and effects of acute attacks therapies. Brain 1994;117:427–34.
64. Goadsby PJ, Edvinsson L. Neuropeptide changes in a case of chronic paroxysmal hemicrania–evidence for trigemino-parasympathetic activation. Cephalagia 1996;16:448–50.
65. Matharu MS, Goadsby PJ. Persistence of attacks of cluster headache after trigeminal nerve root section. Brain 2002;125:976–84.
66. Cohen A. SUN: short lasting unilateral neuralgiform headache attacks. Headache 2017;57(6):1010–20.
67. Eller M, Goadsby PJ. Trigeminal autonomic cephalalgias. Oral Dis 2016;22(1):1–8.
68. Goadsby P. Trigeminal autonomic cephalalgias. Continuum (Minneap Minn) 2012;18(4):883–95.
69. Leone M. Pathophysiology of trigeminal autonomic cephalalgias. Lancet Neurol 2009;8:755–64.
70. Pareja J, Kruszewski P, Sjaastad O. SUNCT syndrome: trials of drugs and anesthetic blockades. Headache 1995;35:138–42.
71. Burns B, Watkins L, Goadsby PJ. Successful treatment of medically intractable cluster headache using occipital nerve stimulation (ONS). Lancet 2007;369(9567):1099–106.
72. Leone M, Proietti Cecchini A, Franzini A, et al. Lessons from 8 years' experience of hypothalamic stimulation in cluster headache. Cephalagia 2008;28(7):787–97.
73. Magis D, Bruno M, Fumal A, et al. Central modulation in cluster headache patients treated with occipital nerve stimulation: an FDG-PET study. BMC Neurol 2011;11:25.
74. Magis D, Schoenen J. Advances and challenges in neurostimulation for headaches. Lancet Neurol 2012;11:708–19.
75. Cohen AS, Matharu MS, Goadsby PJ. Short-lasting unilateral neuralgiform headache attacks with conjunctival injection and tearing (SUNCT) or cranial

autonomic features (SUNA)–A prospective clinical study of SUNCT and SUNA. Brain 2006;129:2746–60.

76. Matharu MS, Cohen AS, Boes CJ, et al. Short-lasting unilateral neuralgiform headache with conjunctival injection and tearing syndrome: a review. Curr Pain Headache Rep 2003;7:308–18.

77. Pareja JA, Cuadrado ML. SUNT syndrome: an update. Expert Opin Pharmacother 2005;6:591–9.

78. Williams MH, Broadley SA. SUNCT and SUNA: clinical features and medical treatment. J Clin Neurosci 2008;15:526–34.

79. Favoni V, Grimaldi D, Pierangeli G, et al. SUNCT/SUNA and neurovascular compression: New cases and critical literature review. Cephalagia 2013;33:1337–48.

80. Goadsby PJ. Trigeminal autonomic cephalalgias. Pathophysiology and classification. Revue Neurol (Paris) 2005;161:692–5.

81. Bartsch T, Falk D, Knudsen K, et al. Deep brain stimulation of the posterior hypothalamic area in intractable short-lasting unilateral neuralgiform headache with conjunctival injection and tearing (SUNCT). Cephalagia 2011;31:1405–8.

82. Chen J, Guo ZY, Yang G, et al. Characterization of neurovascular compression in facial neuralgia patients by 3D high-resolution MRI and image fusion technique. Asian Pac J Trop Med 2012;5:476–9.

83. Cordella R, Franzini A, La Mantia L, et al. Hypothalamic stimulation for trigeminal neuralgia in multiple sclerosis patients: efficacy on the paroxysmal ophthalmic pain. Mult Scler 2009;15:1322–8.

84. Koseoglu E, Daraman Y, Kucuk S, et al. SUNCT syndrome associated with compression of trigeminal nerve. Cephalagia 2005;25:473–5.

85. Lagares A, Gomez PA, Perez-Nunez A, et al. Short-lasting unilateral neuralgiform headache with conjunctival injection and tearing syndrome treated with microvascular decompression of the trigeminal nerve: case report. Neurosurgery 2005;56:E413.

86. Lambru G, Matharu MS. SUNCT and SUNA: medical and surgical treatments. Neurol Sci 2013;34(Suppl 1):S75–81.

87. Lambru G, Matharu MS. SUNCT, SUNA and trigeminal neuralgia: different disorders or variants of the same disorder? Curr Opin Neurol 2014;27:325–31.

88. Lambru G, Shanahan P, Watkins L, et al. Occipital nerve stimulation in the treatment of medically intractable SUNCT and SUNA. Pain physician 2014;17:29–41.

89. Leone M, Franzini A, D'Andrea G, et al. Deep brain stimulation to relieve drug-resistant SUNCT. Ann Neurol 2005;57:924–7.

90. Leone M, Mea E, Genco S, et al. Coexistence of TACS and trigeminal neuralgia: pathophysiological conjectures. Headache 2006;46:1565–70.

91. Miller S, Sinclair A, Davies B, et al. Neurostimulation in the treatment of primary headaches. Pract Neurol 2016;16:362–75.

92. Miller S, Matharu M. Trigeminal autonomic cephalalgias: beyond the conventional treatments. Curr Pain Headache Rep 2014;18(8):438.

93. Morales-Asin F, Espada F, Lopez-Obarrio LA, et al. A SUNCT case with response to surgical treatment. Cephalagia 2000;20:67–8.

94. Cittadini E, Goadsby PJ. Hemicrania continua: a clinical study of 39 patients with diagnostic implications. Brain 2010;133(pt 7):1973–86.

95. Peres MF, Siow HC, Rozen TD. Hemicrania continua with aura. Cephalagia 2002;22(3):246–8.

96. Peres MF, Valencia MM, Goncalves AL. Misdiagnosis of hemicrania continua. Expert Rev Neurother 2009;9(9):1371–8.

97. Prakash S, Shah ND, Chavda BV. Unnecessary extractions in patients with hemicrania continua: case reports and implication for dentistry. J Orofacial pain 2010;24(4):408–11.

98. Viana M, Tassorelli C, Allena M, et al. Diagnostic and therapeutic errors in trigeminal autonomic cephalalgias and hemicrania continua: a systematic review. J Headache Pain 2013;14:14.

99. Delcanho RE, Graff-Radford SB. Chronic paroxysmal hemicrania presenting as a toothache. J orofacial pain 1993;7(3):300–6.

100. Afridi SK, Shields KG, Bhola R, et al. Greater occipital nerve injection in primary headache syndromes-prolonged effects from a single injection. Pain 2006; 122(1–2):126–9.

101. Brighina F, Palermo A, Cosentino G, et al. Prophylaxis of hemicrania continua: two new cases effectively treated with topiramate. Headache 2007;47(3):441–3.

102. Burns B, Watkins L, Goadsby PJ. Treatment of hemicrania continua by occipital nerve stimulation with a novel bion device: long-term follow-up of a crossover study. Lancet Neurol 2008;7(11):1001–12.

103. Camarda C, Camarda R, Monastero R. Chronic paroxysmal hemicrania and hemicrania continua responding to topiramate: two case reports. Clin Neurol Neurosurg 2008;110:88–91.

104. Cohen AS, Goadsby PJ. Paroxysmal hemicrania responding to topiramate. J Neurol Neurosurg Psychiatry 2007;78:96–7.

105. Evers S, Hussedt IW. Alternatives in drug treatment of chronic paroxysmal hemicrania. Headache 1996;36:429–32.

106. Lainez M. Cluster HA and other TACs: pathophysiology and neurostimulation options. Headache 2017;57(2):327–35.

107. Matharu MS, Boes CJ, Goadsby PJ. Management of trigeminal autonomic cephalgias and hemicrania continua. Drugs 2003;63(16):1637–77.

108. May A, Leone M, Afra J, et al. EFNS guidelines on the treatment of cluster headache and other trigeminal-autonomic cephalalgias. Eur J Neurol 2006;13: 1066–77.

109. Sjaastad O, Vincent M. Indomethacin responsive headache syndromes: chronic paroxysmal hemicrania and hemicrania continua. How they were discovered and what we have learned since. Funct Neurol 2010;25(1):49–55.

Sleep and Orofacial Pain

Gary D. Klasser, DMD[a],*, Galit Almoznino, DMD, MSc, MHA[b,c],
Giulio Fortuna, DMD, PhD[d]

KEYWORDS

- Sleep • Sleep disorders • Orofacial pain • Chronic pain • Sleep stages • Screening
- Management strategies

KEY POINTS

- Sleep and pain share a bidirectional relationship.
- Sleep and pain are essential physiologic processes for the survival and continuation of all animal species, from humans to insects.
- Insomnia and chronic orofacial pain conditions involve many common neuroanatomic structures and neurochemical transmitters.
- It is important for practitioners who manage sleep disturbances and/or pain to routinely perform screening procedures for each entity in order that a multidisciplinary approach to management is instituted for enhanced patient care.

INTRODUCTION

Sleep (or at least a physiologic period of quiescence) is a natural physiologic function that is required for survival and continuation of all animal species from insects (fruit flies) to mammals. It is an active neurobehavioral state that is maintained through a highly organized interaction of neurons and neural circuits in the central nervous system (CNS). In humans, it is essential for recovery from fatigue and for tissue repair (eg, heart and skeletal muscles), memory consolidation, and brain function at both the cellular and CNS network levels. Individuals who are totally or partially sleep deprived may develop mood alterations, impaired memory and reduced cognitive abilities, immune system changes, and somatic pain-related complaints.[1,2] This is considered

Disclosure: The authors have nothing to disclose.
[a] Department of Diagnostic Sciences, Louisiana State University Health Sciences Center, School of Dentistry, 1100 Florida Avenue, Box 140, New Orleans, LA 70119, USA; [b] Department of Oral Medicine, Sedation and Maxillofacial Imaging, Orofacial Sensory Clinic, Hebrew University-Hadassah School of Dental Medicine, PO Box 91120, Jerusalem, Israel; [c] Division of Big Data, Department of Community Dentistry, Orofacial Sensory Clinic, Hebrew University-Hadassah School of Dental Medicine, PO Box 91120, Jerusalem, Israel; [d] Department of Neurosciences, Reproductive and Odontostomatological Sciences, Federico II University of Naples, Via Pansini, 5, Naples 80131, Italy
* Corresponding author.
E-mail address: gklass@lsuhsc.edu

Dent Clin N Am 62 (2018) 629–656
https://doi.org/10.1016/j.cden.2018.06.005

nonrestorative sleep because it commonly refers to the unrefreshed feeling on awakening and is present in approximately 10% of the general population.[1,3]

In order to classify and describe sleep disorders, the American Academy of Sleep Medicine developed the International Classification of Sleep Disorders, Third edition (ICSD-3).[4] ICSD-3 includes 7 major categories: insomnia, sleep-related breathing disorders, central disorders of hypersomnia, circadian rhythm sleep-wake disorders, parasomnias, sleep-related movement disorders, and other sleep disorders.[4] The ICSD-3 divides these 7 major categories into 60 diagnoses, and it also includes an appendix for classification of sleep disorders associated with medical and neurologic disorders.[4]

Overall, in most adults, sleep onset normally occurs within 20 to 30 minutes after the individual goes to bed and sleep typically endures for 6 to 9 hours. However, there is considerable individual variation as a result of different sleep habits, employment requirements, and so forth.

Sleep is customarily divided into 2 distinct categories: non–rapid eye movement (NREM) and rapid eye movement (REM) sleep (**Table 1**). During a typical night, there are 3 to 5 NREM to REM cycles (ultradian rhythm cycle), with each cycle having a duration of approximately 90 to 120 minutes. NREM sleep is further divided into 3 distinct stages based on electroencephalogram (EEG) activity: Stages N1 and N2 (lighter stages of the sleep cycle) and stage N3 (formerly called stages 3 and 4, which is dominated by slow wave brain activity, or slow wave sleep [SWS]). REM sleep, often referred to as Paradoxical sleep, because all skeletal muscles are in a hypotonic state, as if the body is paralyzed, involves high activity in the CNS and autonomic nervous system. Normal sleep has an oscillatory rhythm

Table 1
Normal sleep of young adult

Sleep Stage	Time in Sleep Stage (%)	Sleep Characteristics
Relaxed wakefulness (stage W)	<5	Alpha + beta activity (neural oscillations ranging from 7.5 to 12.5 Hz + from 12.5 to 30 Hz)
NREM		High-amplitude/low-frequency activity + decreased muscle tone with slow rolling eye movements
Stage 1 (transitional) N1	2–5	Alpha activity gradually decreases (presleep 8–12 Hz) + theta activity (4–8 Hz) appears, the eyes move slowly + muscle activity slows
Stage 2 (sleep onset) N2	45–55	[a]Spindle waves (7–14 Hz) + [b]K-complexes appear on EEG, body temperature decreases + heart rate slows
Stage 3 (slow wave)	3–8	Delta/slow wave activity (1–4 Hz) starts to dominate the EEG
Stage 4 (slow wave)	10–15	
REM (stage R)	20–25	Low-voltage fast activity (beta + theta waves), muscle hypotonia, dreaming, brain activity with rapid eye movements

Note: stage 3 + 4 now considered N3.
Abbreviations: EEG, electroencephalogram; Hz, Hertz.
[a] Spindle waves: (burstlike trains of waves in the 11-Hz to 16-Hz range with a total duration ≥0.5 seconds).
[b] K-complexes: well-defined biphasic waves lasting greater than or equal to 0.5 seconds and usually maximal over the frontal cortex.

whereby it fluctuates from active periods to quiet periods. These alternating active (phase A) and quiet (phase B) sleep periods reflect the cyclic alternating pattern (CAP) of electrocortical events that recur at regular intervals. During these CAP periods there are frequent sleep arousals or microarousals whereby structures such as the brain, cardiac, and muscle tissues undergo reactivations (each lasting 3–15 seconds) within the active periods. Arousals are the response of the sleeping brain to external (environmental) and internal (physiologic or pathologic) stimuli. The purpose of these arousals or active periods are that they are "windows" whereby sleeping individuals can readjust their body positions, reset body temperature, and, if any harmful event is perceived, can become fully awake; that is, a fight-or-flight reaction could be triggered. In normal healthy adults, sleep arousals occur between 7 and 15 times per hour of sleep and tend to occur at the end of an NREM period.

The International Association for the Study of Pain defines pain as "an unpleasant sensory and emotional experience associated with actual or potential tissue damage, or described in terms of such damage."[5] This definition is currently being scrutinized and a revised version stating that "Pain is a distressing experience associated with actual or potential tissue damage with sensory, emotional, cognitive, and social components"[6] has been proposed. A more pragmatic definition to consider is that chronic pain is pain that extends beyond the period of tissue healing and/or with low levels of identified disorder that are insufficient to explain the presence and/or extent of the pain. Overall, pain should be recognized as a complex interaction of cognitive, affective, and sensory processes making it a personal experience. Orofacial pain, which may be a form of chronic pain, includes a heterogeneous group of conditions, such as dental, mucosal, musculoskeletal, neurovascular, and neuropathic pains.[7]

Simplistically, acute and chronic pain were separated by temporal discrimination whereby acute pain was considered pain lasting 3 months or less and pain was considered chronic when it lasts or recurs for more than 3 to 6 months.[5] Acute pain is biologically adaptive because it creates hypervigilance to warn the individual of potential tissue damage or as a response to injury and is necessary for species survival. Contrarily, chronic pain is not biologically adaptive per se and, because of this, such pain becomes the sole or predominant clinical problem in some patients. Chronic pain may persist despite successful management of the conditions that initially caused it, or because the underlying medical condition cannot be treated successfully. However, chronic pain syndromes currently are not represented in the International Classification of Diseases in a systematic manner. Therefore, a new phenomenological definition, created because the cause is unknown for many forms of chronic pain, has been proposed (**Box 1**).

Box 1
Proposed classification of chronic primary pain for the International Classification of Diseases 11

Chronic primary pain is chronic pain in 1 or more anatomic regions that is characterized by significant emotional distress (anxiety, anger/frustration, or depressed mood) and functional disability (interference in daily life activities and reduced participation in social roles). Chronic primary pain is multifactorial: biological, psychological, and social factors contribute to the pain syndrome. The diagnosis is appropriate independently of identified biological or psychological contributors unless another diagnosis would better account for the presenting symptoms. Specific diagnoses to be considered are chronic cancer pain, chronic postsurgical or posttraumatic pain, chronic neuropathic pain, chronic headache or orofacial pain, chronic visceral pain, and chronic musculoskeletal pain.

The interrelationship between pain and sleep is complex and it may seem that pain and sleep should have a minimal influence on one another because pain is a conscious process, whereas sleep is a state whereby awareness of the surrounding environment decreases and the neural networks related to wakefulness become subdued. Nevertheless, pain can intrude into the goal-directed behavior of sleep, bringing pain into consciousness, thereby disturbing sleep, whereas poor sleep can prevent adequate physiologic and psychological restoration and refreshment, thus contributing to enhanced pain. Ultimately, this bidirectional relationship can develop into a vicious cycle. In a large (n = 2406) survey that investigated the relationship between sleep and pain, it was reported that 61% (n = 1468) of the study participants reported pain in the 3 months preceding the survey. The prevalence of sleep disturbances either alone or in combination with pain was 50% (n = 1203). It was also found that 58% of the respondents reporting a pain problem also had a sleep problem, whereas 70% of respondents reporting a sleep problem also had a pain problem.[8]

EPIDEMIOLOGY OF SLEEP AND PAIN

Most young adults average between 7 and 8 hours of sleep nightly, but there is a significant individual and night-to-night variability. It seems that the strongest factor that influences sleep continuity and the distribution of sleep stages through the night is that of chronologic age. The sleep pattern of newborn infants dramatically differs from that of adults. During the first year of life, infants sleep twice as much as adults and, unlike adults, enter sleep through REM. NREM-REM cycles, controlled by the ultradian process, are present at birth, at a frequency of 50-minute to 60-minute cycle periods in newborns, which are of shorter duration than the approximately 90-minute to 120-minute periods in adults. SWS is not present at birth but develops by the age of 2 to 6 months. The amount of SWS steadily declines from maximal levels in the young to almost nonexistent amounts in the elderly. Interestingly, the need to sleep does not decrease with advancing age; what changes in the elderly is the ability to maintain sleep. Sleep insufficiency exists when sleep is insufficient to support adequate alertness, performance, and health, either because of reduced total sleep time (decreased quantity) or fragmentation of sleep by brief arousals (decreased quality).[4] It is associated with both morbidity and mortality, such as motor vehicle accidents, industrial disasters, medical errors, and other occupational errors.[9] Persons experiencing sleep insufficiency are also more likely to have chronic diseases such as hypertension, diabetes, depression, and obesity, as well as cancer, reduced quality of life, and productivity.[9] Acute sleep deprivation refers to no sleep or a reduction in the usual total sleep time, usually lasting 1 or 2 days. Chronic sleep insufficiency (also called sleep restriction) exists when an individual routinely sleeps less than the amount required for optimal functioning. The cause of sleep insufficiency may be a broad scale of societal factors such as 24-hour access to technology and work schedules, but sleep disorders such as insomnia (a disorder that involves delayed sleep onset or difficulty maintaining sleep) or obstructive sleep apnea (OSA) also play an important role.[9] It is estimated that 50 to 70 million US adults have sleep or wakefulness disorders.[9]

Data from the 2009 Behavioral Risk Factor Surveillance System Sleep module in the United States were used to assess the prevalence of unhealthy sleep behaviors by selected sociodemographic factors and geographic variations in 12 states (Table 2). The analysis determined that, among 74,571 adult respondents in 12 states, 35.3% reported less than 7 hours of sleep during a typical 24-hour period, 48.0% reported snoring, 37.9% reported unintentionally falling asleep during the day at least once in the preceding month, and 4.7% reported nodding off or falling asleep while

Table 2
Adults reporting selected sleep behaviors in 12 states using the Behavioral Risk Factor Surveillance System, United States, 2009

Age (y)	Unintentionally Fell Asleep During Day at Least Once in the Past Month (%)	Nodded off or Fell Asleep While Driving in the Past Month (%)
18 to <25	43.7	4.5
25 to <35	36.1	7.2
35 to <45	34.0	5.7
45 to <55	35.3	3.9
55 to <65	36.5	3.1
≥65	44.6	2.0
Race/Ethnicity		
White non-Hispanic	33.4	3.2
Black non-Hispanic	52.4	6.5
Hispanic	41.9	6.3
Other non-Hispanic	41.0	7.2
Sex		
Male	38.4	5.8
Female	37.3	3.5

From Centers for Disease Control and Prevention. Unhealthy sleep-related behaviors - 12 states, 2009. Morb Mortal Wkly Rep 2011;60(8):232–8.

driving at least once in the preceding month.[10] Using data from 2 consecutive survey cycles (2005–2006 and 2007–2008), which included 10,896 respondents aged greater than or equal to 20 years, it was reported by the National Health and Nutrition Examination Survey that a short sleep duration was more common among adults aged 20 to 39 years (37.0%) or 40 to 59 years (40.3%) than among adults aged greater than or equal to 60 years (32.0%), and among non-Hispanic black people (53.0%) compared with non-Hispanic white people (34.5%), Mexican-Americans (35.2%), or those of other race/ethnicity (41.7%). In addition, adults who reported sleeping less than the recommended 7 to 9 hours per night were more likely to have difficulty performing many daily tasks.[10,11]

As previously described, individuals who experience chronic pain commonly also report sleep disturbance as a clinical symptom, with 50% to 90% of people with pain reporting sleep disturbances of some description, with insomnia being the most common problem.[12]

Epidemiologic studies have shown that orofacial pain is prevalent in the general population, at around 17% to 26% (excluding dental pain), of which 7% to 11% is of a chronic nature.[13] In patients experiencing acute and/or chronic orofacial pain (COFP), whereby the pain involves the head and neck area and includes such disorders as temporomandibular disorders (muscle and/or joint), neuropathic pain, and neurovascular pain disorders, disturbed sleep is commonly problematic. A cross-sectional population-based study of 4000 individuals found that patients with orofacial pain had a relative risk of 3.7 for a high level of sleep disturbance.[14] Furthermore, it has been reported that pain-related awakening occurs in about one-third of patients with persistent orofacial pain and this is significantly correlated with self-reported pain intensity.[15] It is noteworthy that the development of chronic pain coincides with the development of sleep disturbance, and vice versa. Furthermore, both chronic pain and sleep disturbances share an array of comorbidities, such as obesity, type 2 diabetes, depression, and other conditions (discussed later).[16,17]

INTERRELATIONSHIP BETWEEN SLEEP AND PAIN

In order for humans to survive and flourish, they require both pain and sleep. However, chronic impairments in the systems regulating sleep and pain can have a broad negative impact on health and well-being. During normal sleep in healthy adults, nociceptive transmission is partially attenuated to preserve sleep continuity, with a higher threshold or lower response rate to noxious stimuli in light sleep (stages N1 and N2) that becomes more important with deep-stage sleep (stage N3) and becomes variable in REM sleep. Sensory transmission in general is attenuated during sleep such that low-intensity stimuli may have little or no effect on sleep quality when healthy individuals are sleeping in conditions favoring good sleep quality (eg, a quiet, comfortable environment).[18]

In a recent critical narrative review to identify trends suggestive of directionality among sleep and pain, the following was reported: (1) there is an indication that sleep disturbance increases the risk for new-onset cases of chronic pain in pain-free individuals; (2) sleep disturbances worsen the long-term prognosis of existing headache and chronic musculoskeletal pain; and (3) sleep disturbances have an influence on daily fluctuations in clinical pain. Furthermore, good sleep seems to improve the long-term prognosis of individuals with tension-type headache, migraine, and chronic musculoskeletal pain. On further analysis, the investigators concluded that there seems to be a trend that sleep impairments present a stronger, more reliable predictor of pain than pain is of sleep impairments.[19] A possible mechanism for this finding may be that altered sleep decreases pain thresholds, thus resulting in increased sensitivity to pain.[19]

Overall, pain and sleep interactions may be viewed from the perspective of both linear and circular models. During acute pain, the influence of pain on sleep is usually of short duration; this follows a "linear model" whereby pain precedes poor sleep and sleep returns to normalcy once the acute pain is resolved. However, in patients with chronic pain, a "circular model" often predominates in as much as a night of poor sleep is followed by a day with more intense and variable pain, which is then followed by a night of nonrestorative sleep and morning-related complaints of unrefreshed sleep. Therefore, it seems that pain, specifically when chronic, can trigger poor sleep quality and disrupt its restorative benefit.[18]

NEUROBIOLOGY OF SLEEP AND PAIN
Neuroanatomic Structures and Functional Changes

In patients with chronic pain, central and peripheral mechanisms involving neuroplastic changes have been well documented and are described as the pain neuromatrix.[20] This neuromatrix is thought to be a widely distributed brain neural matrix that involves neuroanatomic structures that include the primary and secondary somatosensory cortex, the insula, cingulate cortex, thalamus, and limbic areas. Of further note, chronic pain conditions result in atrophy of the medial prefrontal cortex (mPFC), the hippocampus, and the anterior cingulated cortex (ACC).[21] Decreased activation of the prefrontal cortex (PFC) has been hypothesized to result in a reduction of inhibitory drive to the limbic system and consequently in its overactivity resulting in an alteration in the modulation of pain.[22] Activation in the mPFC is positively correlated with activation in the hippocampal complex, an area that seems to have a role in pain augmentation in pain-free individuals.

The literature on structural and functional changes in the CNS of individuals with sleep disturbances is limited. Notwithstanding, there are a few structural MRI studies of individuals with chronic insomnia, but the results have been contradictory. In a pilot study by Riemann and colleagues,[23] hippocampal structures, measured by volume, were atrophied. Contrarily, in a similar study, it was reported that there was a decrease in PFC size (specifically orbital-frontal cortex) without any decreases in hippocampal volume.[24] In one of the first large-scale studies addressing structural changes in the insomnia brain, statistically significant changes in brain volume were not found, although there was a trend toward hippocampal shrinkage.[25] Notwithstanding the inconsistency of these results, insomnia may be correlated with similar changes in brain structures to those documented in individuals with chronic pain.

In the few studies that have addressed functional brain changes in individuals with insomnia, these studies found increases in glucose metabolism during various sleep stages, with increased metabolism in the amygdala, hippocampus, ACC, and mPFC when contrasted with healthy controls.[24] This increase in activation has been hypothesized to reflect persistent sensory processing, which in turn contributes to a shallower sleep. During wakeful states, people with insomnia show decreased metabolism in the PFC, similar to that reported in the brains of depressed individuals. It is hypothesized that this decrease contributes to the increase of limbic activity through a process of disinhibition similar to that observed in chronic pain.

Neurotransmitters Involved in Sleep and Pain

Potential mechanisms for the bidirectional relationship between chronic pain and sleep disturbances may involve the following processes: central neuroimmune activation, disturbed neurotransmitter balance, and neuroendocrine axis aberrations. Imbalances in central proinflammatory and antiinflammatory cytokines have been detected across several chronic pain populations, and these cytokines, especially interleukin (IL)-1b and tumor necrosis factor alpha (TNF-α), play a role in sleep regulation and homeostasis.[26] Levels of IL-1b and TNF-α vary with the sleep-wake cycle, and, in animal models, administration of IL-1b and TNF-α increases NREM sleep in a dose-dependent and time-dependent manner. IL-1b typically causes sleep fragmentation, high doses suppress both REM and NREM sleep, and sleep deprivation has been shown to increase IL-1b messenger RNA in the brain.[27] In experimental chronic pain models, CNS cytokines have been suggested to be pivotal mediators involved in neuroimmune activation pathways and neuroinflammation, driving the transition from acute to chronic pain.[26] Across a variety of chronic pain states of varying causes, some cross-sectional studies have revealed evidence of increased cerebrospinal fluid (CSF) levels of proinflammatory cytokines TNF-α, IL-1b, IL-6, and IL-8.[26] Also, in complex regional pain syndrome, decreased levels of antiinflammatory cytokines IL-4 and IL-10 are reported.[26]

There are many neurotransmitters involved with both pain mechanisms and sleep regulation. Some of the more prominent neurotransmitters involved in sleep and pain interactions are discussed here. Serotonin (5-hydroxytryptamine [5-HT]) is a mediator linking sleep and pain because this neurotransmitter is involved in descending pain modulation pathways, affective disorders, and regulation of NREM sleep. In animal models, REM sleep deprivation has been shown to decrease levels of 5-HT in the frontal cortex and hippocampus[28] and, interestingly, decreased concentrations of 5-HT, dopamine, and norepinephrine metabolites have been found in the CSF of patients with fibromyalgia.[29] Serotonin exerts complex modulatory effects on nociceptive transmission in the spinal dorsal horn, and, depending on type and duration of pain, both pronociceptive and antinociceptive effects can be observed. When 5-HT binds to postsynaptic 5-HT$_{1A}$, or presynaptic 5-HT$_{1B/D}$ receptors, pain-inhibitory effects are achieved through diminished excitability of spinothalamic neurons, excitatory interneurons, and inhibited neurotransmitter release from primary afferents.[30] However, if levels of 5-HT are decreased because of sleep disturbance interactions, then the possibility of a disinhibition of descending inhibitory pain pathways may occur, resulting in pathophysiologic alterations leading to an enhancement of central sensitization, which has been implicated in several chronic pain states. Another emerging body of research suggests a role for altered dopaminergic signaling in the connection between disturbed sleep and chronic pain, possibly contributing to dysregulation of wakefulness and disrupted sleep continuity.[19]

Gamma-aminobutyric acid (GABA) is another neurotransmitter that interacts with sleep and pain. GABA is an inhibitory neurotransmitter and functions on GABA receptors located in the anterior hypothalamus. GABA is also an important neurotransmitter involved with the sleep-wake cycle. Activity of GABAergic cells in the ventrolateral preoptic nucleus (VLPO) in the anterior hypothalamus is implicated in production of NREM sleep, whereas the GABAergic cells in the area adjacent to the VLPO are thought to promote REM sleep by inhibiting the noradrenergic neurons located in the locus coeruleus and serotonergic neurons in the dorsal raphe nucleus REM-off nuclei of the brainstem.[31] In addition, GABA release in the thalamus mediates the thalamic sensory filter to filter out sensory input coming to the thalamus from spinal and trigeminal ascending transmission. If there is deficient GABAergic neurotransmission during sleep, the filter effect is reduced, allowing ascending sensory input to pass through the thalamic filter, affecting the cortex and causing hyperarousal as might occur with a barrage of nociceptive input associated with chronic pain.[32]

Orexins (also called hypocretins) are 2 neuropeptides (orexin-A and orexin-B) with key roles in regulation of arousal and metabolism with possible involvement in pain signaling and/or modulation. These compounds bind to their corresponding receptors (OX-1 and OX-2) throughout the brain and spinal cord in accordance with circadian rhythmic control of orexin levels (through suprachiasmatic nuclei input), with their concentration being highest during the waking period. Orexin levels also increase during a period of forced sleep deprivation. It remains unclear whether this increase during sleep deprivation represents orexin opposing and attempting to override the sleep drive or producing a stress response to sleep deprivation.[33] With regard to pain signaling/modulation, it has been reported in a rodent model that orexin activates intracellular calcium signaling through a protein kinase C–dependent pathway that may be involved in pain modulation.[34] Holland and Goadsby,[35] in a study involving orexin- A and orexin-B, reported that orexin-B had no effect on trigeminal firing but orexin-A played a key inhibitory role in trigeminal responses.

In addition, experimental studies have shown that sleep deprivation may inhibit synthesis of endogenous opioids, downregulate central opioid receptors, and also reduce the affinity for specific opioid receptors, which might reduce the analgesic efficacy of exogenously administered opioids, but further mechanistic research is warranted.[19] Two well-designed studies in human healthy volunteers and patients with chronic temporomandibular joint disorder have shown that impaired descending pain-inhibitory function associated with disrupted sleep might be a pivotal mechanism linking sleep and pain.[36,37] This finding implies that it is likely that undisrupted sleep continuity, and/or undisturbed sleep architecture, is of great importance for the function of the endogenous descending pain modulatory systems and potentially also for the action of exogenous analgesics.

INFLUENCE OF PAIN ON SLEEP STAGES

Sleep can be highly impaired by pain, mainly chronic pain, and poor sleep can have a negative impact on pain perception and quality. In a study using gradual increase in temperature to produce noxious stimuli during the various stages of sleep, it was necessary for a greater amount of thermal stimulation be produced to induce arousal from SWS and REM sleep than from N2 sleep, and temperatures that induced arousal from SWS and REM sleep were close to the pain tolerance observed during wakefulness.[38] This finding implies that both those phases of sleep (N3 and REM) are more refractory to painful thermal stimuli than N2 and that the intensity of noxious stimulus plays a pivotal role in the disruption of the various sleep stages.[38] These results were consistent with another study on polygraphic responses to cool (24°C), warm (37°C), and heat pain (>46°C) stimuli applied to shoulder skin during different sleep stages, showing that heat pain stimuli were capable of inducing more sleep arousal than the other two stimuli and that such arousals were greater in the lighter sleep stages (48.3%) than in the deeper stages (27.9%).[39]

In addition, a painful stimulus in N2 was followed by a high-amplitude negative wave with typical features of a K complex,[40] which might be interpreted as an attempt of the brain to induce arousal from the sleep state. These K complex intrusions seem to be associated with fatigue, pain, and nonrestorative sleep in patients with fibromyalgia,[32] as well as an increase in alpha-wave activity.[41] This intrusion of alpha wave during SWS would cause a shift in sleep pattern, a decrease in total sleep time, and an increase in hyperalgesia. In contrast, an increase of spindles in the EEG might be considered a way to prevent the disruption of sleep by pain and therefore would act as a gate control to inhibit ascending painful stimuli in reaching the cortex and causing arousal.[32]

CHRONIC OROFACIAL PAIN AND SLEEP DISORDERS

As previously discussed, there exists a complex bidirectional relationship between chronic pain and sleep, with similar principles applying to chronic pain emanating from the orofacial region.[42] Detailed descriptions for the various primary headaches can be found in Robert W. Mier and Shuchi Dhadwal's article, "Primary Headaches," in this issue.

Headache

The relationship between headache and sleep disturbances is complex and extensive. Although cause and effect are yet to be established, headache and sleep disturbances share common neurophysiologic and anatomic substrates, suggesting a bidirectional influence.

These mutual interactions are mediated by time (headache may be a symptom of a sleep disturbance and occur during sleep, after sleep, and in relationship with sleep stages) or by quantitative (excess, lack, poor quality, or short duration of sleep can cause a headache) relationships; therefore, these conditions may influence each other and may represent a risk for one another.

Migraine

This type of headache may be accompanied by different types of sleep problems, such as poor quality of sleep and parasomnias. Interestingly, sleep can be both a trigger and cure for migraine. In a large study (n = 2695), patients with migraine (45.5%) had insufficient sleep more than those with nonmigraine headache (32.9%)

or nonheadache (20.4%).[43] It seems that patients with migraine have insomnia more than controls and that migrainous attacks are more severe in patients with migraine than in those with probable migraine (PM), although no difference was found between patients with migraine and those with PM in terms of prevalence of insomnia.[44] Insomnia is therefore the most common sleep disturbance in patients with chronic migraine (CM), and it is more frequent and severe than in patients with episodic migraine (EM).[45]

Migraine has also been associated with sleep-related breathing disorders (SBDs) and sleep-related movement disorder, specifically, sleep-related bruxism (SRB). In a study performed on 3411 patients, the cumulative incidence of developing migraine during the follow-up was higher in the SBD cohort than in the control group, higher in men than in women with SBD, and higher in middle-aged adults (20–64 years old).[46] Contrarily, a systematic review reported that SRB in adults is more prevalent in patients with CM by 3.8 times,[47] whereas another study failed to find any relationship between migraine with and without aura and SRB.[48] In patients with EM, there was an increased sleepiness compared with a control group without migraine, as well as in CM.[49]

Tension-type headache

Tension-type headache (TTH) is the most common form of primary headache in the general population, with the most common sleep problem being insomnia.[50] In a study of 570 patients presenting with TTH, insomnia was present in 13.2% of the patients with TTH compared with 5.8% without TTH.[50] A subcohort of patients with TTH fulfilling the criteria for PM showed the same prevalence of insomnia as those patients without PM.[50] However, there are conflicting data regarding the relationship between TTH and SBD, mainly OSA. Chiu and colleagues[51] reported a higher prevalence of TTH among patients with OSA with a higher chance for this type of patient to develop TTH, whereas a different study failed to show any significant association between OSA and TTH.[52] TTH has also been associated with sleep-related movement disorder, mainly SRB, whereby adults have a 3-fold increase for the risk of developing TTH.[47]

Trigeminal autonomic cephalalgias

The most common sleep disorder associated with cluster headache (CH) is OSA, whose prevalence in patients with CH seems to be as high as 6 in 10, with patients with CH being 8.4 times more likely to exhibit OSA than normal individuals.[53] Another investigation confirmed an association between CH and OSA but only in the CH episode and not in the CH interval, and also showed that OSA is more severe in chronic than in episodic CH and that patients with CH may not only have obstructive apneas but also central apneas.[54]

It has also been hypothesized that an association between CH attacks and REM sleep exists, because some patients awakened by CH attacks at night remembered dreams and that those attacks occurred about 1 to 2 hours after falling asleep, more or less when REM sleep should occur.[53] However, data are still conflicting; one study showed that an association was found between episodic CH and REM sleep but not between chronic CH and REM sleep,[55] whereas another failed to show any association between episodic CH attacks and REM sleep.[56]

Painful Cranial Neuropathies

Painful cranial neuropathies (detailed description can be found in Janina Christoforou's article, "Neuropathic Orofacial Pain," in this issue) are a group of disorders characterized by pain in the head-neck region mediated by various nerves, whose dysfunction and/or dysregulation lead to various neurologic conditions.

Trigeminal neuralgia

Trigeminal neuralgia (TN) has been associated with sleep disturbances in some cases. One investigation showed that 31% of patients with TN often awoke at night with TN attacks, 30% had attacks occasionally, and only 22% never experienced attacks at night.[57] In another study, 50% of patients with TN were awakened from sleep by pain while experiencing an overall poor quality of sleep.[58]

Painful trigeminal neuropathy

The 2 most common forms of painful trigeminal neuropathy (PTN) are postherpetic trigeminal neuralgia (PHTN) and painful posttraumatic trigeminal neuropathy (PPTN). In patients with PHTN, heterogeneous sensory abnormalities and different types/levels of unrelenting pain are usually present, whose severity is significantly influenced by the combination of multiple psychophysiologic factors, including sleep disturbances. Coincidently, high-intensity pain can be considered the strongest risk factor for insomnia, which was moderate to severe in about 30% of patients with PHTN.[59] This correlation between pain intensity and sleep disturbances has been confirmed by studies on pharmacologic treatment of pain in PHTN, in which reduction in pain intensity resulted in an overall sleep improvement.[60] However, studies with polysomnography have shown that patients with PHTN not only have sleep reduction and fragmentation but also reduction in N3 and REM sleep.[42]

Patients with PPTN may experience sleep disturbances similarly to TN and other neuropathic pain,[58] with a chance of waking up from sleep 4 times greater than a control group.[42]

Burning mouth syndrome

This condition has been associated not only with several medical unexplained symptoms but also with sleep problems compared with controls.[61] Several investigation have highlighted the relationship between burning mouth syndrome (BMS) and sleep, reporting a frequency ranging from 67.1%[62] to 80%[63,64] with an increased risk of about 3-fold of developing BMS for patients with sleep disorders, whereas it was 4 times higher for female patients.[65] The analyses performed with specific self-administered questionnaires (Pittsburgh Sleep Quality Index [PSQI]; Epworth Sleepiness Scale [ESS]) for sleep disturbances, showed that patients with BMS have poorer sleep quality than controls with a positive correlation to anxious and depressed mood.[62-64] Therefore, sleep dysfunction may be a risk factor for BMS and may represent a possible target for treatment.[61]

Temporomandibular Disorders

Temporomandibular disorder (TMD) is a broad term, which includes a group of musculoskeletal conditions affecting the craniofacial masticatory system and the temporomandibular joint (TMJ). Researchers studying TMD tend to group together patients with muscular and skeletal alterations, which indicates its complexity through the presence of comorbidities, as well as with sleep disturbances.[66] On PSQI total score, poor sleep was statistically significant in patients with TMD compared with a control group[66,67] with a worse sleep quality component of the PSQI questionnaire in one study[66] and with more sleep dysfunction and poorer sleep duration in another.[67] Similar results were found on ESS; patients with myofascial pain experienced excessive daytime sleepiness more frequently than controls.[68]

In a large cohort of initially TMD-free adults followed prospectively, subjective sleep quality deteriorated progressively before the onset of pain symptoms in patients who developed painful TMD, the investigators hypothesizing that poor sleep quality might have a hyperalgesic effect, thereby resulting in a higher risk of developing TMD.[69]

However, these data on sleep disturbance and TMD based on self-report sleep measures must be interpreted with caution, because little concordance between PSQI scores and polysomnography indicators were found.[70] It seems that poor sleep quality in TMD was better accounted for by symptoms of depression than by myofascial pain or sleep disturbance as recorded by objective sleep measures, such as polysomnography.[70]

Temporomandibular joint disorders

In sleep deprived mice, the TMJ synovial membrane showed greater vessel hyperplasia and condylar cartilage hypertrophy. In addition, inflammatory factors IL-1β, TNF-α, and the bone metabolism-related factor RANKL (receptor activator of nuclear factor kappa-B ligand) was increased in condylar cartilage.[71] In addition, sleep deprivation in rats seems to activate the ERK (extracellular receptor kinase) pathway responsible for TMJ destruction by promoting the expression of metalloproteinases (MMPs), MMP-1, MMP-3, and MMP-13.[72]

Despite the fact that, in mouse models, sleep deprivation is able to cause an increase in plasma levels of estradiol,[73] which aggravates TMJ inflammation through the nuclear factor kappa-B (NF-κB) pathway, leading to the induction of proinflammatory cytokines,[74] a study performed on 45 women failed to show any significant association between the pattern of sleep quality and the presence of degenerative changes of the TMJ ($P = .36$).[75]

Masticatory and cervical muscle disorders

Animal models have shown that sleep deprivation may alter the expression of myosin heavy chain isoforms of masseter muscle fibers[76] and promote the presence of acute inflammatory cells, congested vessels, fibrosis, and high cellularity in the masseter and temporalis muscle fibers,[77] thereby contributing to the pathogenesis of TMD. It has been shown that the prevalence of moderate to severe sleep disturbance was significantly higher in a myofascial pain group than in the control group.[78]

The most common sleep disorders in patients with myofascial pain are insomnia, OSA, and SRB. A longitudinal (10 years) study reported that the risk of developing myofascial pain was double in patients with insomnia compared with controls.[79] Similar results (arousals associated with all types of respiratory events) using polysomnography were obtained in a cohort of patients already with a diagnosis of myofascial pain.[80]

More complicated and controversial seems to be the relationship between SRB and myofascial pain. Some studies have shown that self-reported SRB occurred significantly more often in patients with TMD, who reported more temporalis muscle activity possibly related to SRB.[81] It also seems that painful TMD is related to both awake and sleep bruxism, which are dependently associated and interact additively, whereby each factor amplifies the effect of the other.[82]

However, although self-reported rates of SRB were significantly higher in cases versus controls, polysomnography-based studies failed to show that myofascial pain can be explained by increased numbers of SRB episodes per hour of sleep or decreased time between SRB events.[83] Therefore, it was suggested that consideration be given to abandoning the notion that SRB is a causal factor for myofascial TMD.[84] A recent systematic review showed that there is a high correlation between

TMD and SRB; however, the level of evidence was low to moderate because of short-comings among the various study designs.[85]

SCREENING FOR SLEEP DISORDERS IN OROFACIAL PAIN

Screening for sleep disorders is recommended in patients with COFP at their first appointment and during follow-up visits. An algorithm for screening and monitoring of patients with sleep disorders and COFP is presented in **Figs. 1** and **2**.

Diagnostic work-up of patients with COFP should combine assessment of COFP history and patterns relative to the sleep/wake cycle.[7] Sleep and pain diaries should be maintained and evaluated for at least a few weeks in order to monitor the frequency and variations of COFP and sleep. It is essential to collect information from partners, caretakers, and parents (for child patients) concerning sleep habits, exaggerated daytime sleepiness, restless sleep, periodic limb movements, teeth grinding, TMJ noise, snoring, witnessed apneas, substance use (eg, alcohol, tobacco, caffeine), and other habits (see **Fig. 1**).

A medical history and physical examination should be performed to determine whether the sleep disorder is related to another medical and/or psychiatric disorder, prescribed medications, drug and alcohol abuse, and/or poor lifestyle. Complex medical status may result from or may coexist with sleep disorders, with a higher prevalence in patients with cardiac disease, hypertension, diabetes, peptic ulcers,

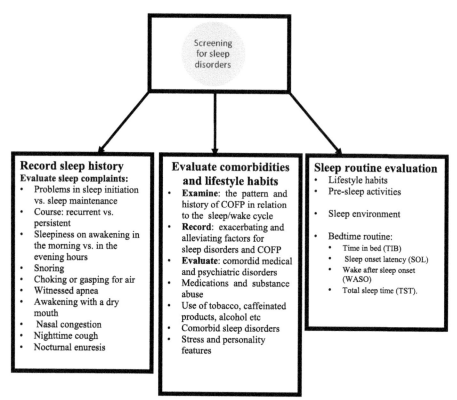

Fig. 1. Identifying and monitoring sleep disorders in patients with COFP. (*Adapted from* Al-moznino G, Haviv Y, Sharav Y, et al. An update of management of insomnia in patients with chronic orofacial pain. Oral Dis 2017;23:1045; with permission.)

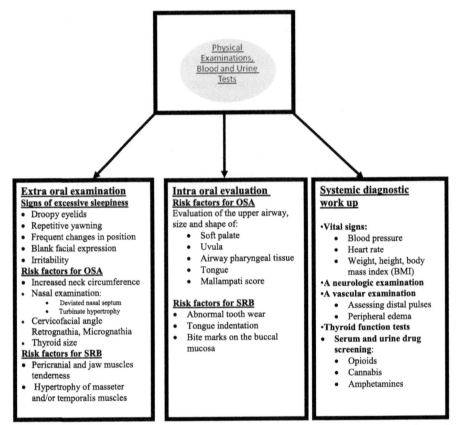

Fig. 2. Physical examinations, blood and urine tests as part of the diagnostic work-up of sleep disorders in patients with COFP. BMI, body mass index.

arthritis, asthma, neurologic problems, and menstrual problems.[86] Furthermore, sleep deprivation may be a result of medications routinely used to treat COFP, particularly when substance abuse is present.[42]

Risk factors for OSA (obesity, specific craniofacial morphologies such as narrow jaw, retrognathia, and increased neck circumference) and for SRB (pericranial and jaw muscle tenderness as well as signs of hypertrophy of masseter and/or temporalis muscles) should be assessed (see **Fig. 2**). Intraoral examination should record oropharyngeal structures; for example, palatal height, tongue and tonsil size, and Mallampati score (for OSA screening), as well as abnormal tooth wear, tongue indentation, and ridgelike bite marks inside the cheek (for SRB screening) (see **Fig. 2**).

Validated sleep measurements should be used, such as visual or numeric analog scales, or sleep questionnaires such as the PSQI, Insomnia severity index, BEARS (Bedtime, Excessive Daytime Sleepiness, Awakening During the Night, Regularity and Duration of Sleep, Snoring) (used in the pediatric population) or STOP-BANG (Snoring, Tired, Observed, Pressure, Body Mass Index, Age, Neck size, Gender) sleep screening tool, ESS, and a wide variety of other questionnaires reviewed elsewhere.[87]

Additional diagnostic examinations should be used as needed, including full-night polysomnographic study, actigraphy, EEG, electro-oculogram, electromyogram (EMG), and neuroimaging.[87–91] The choice of the specific tool primarily depends on the interest of the clinician and whether the intention is to collect objective or subjective data concerning sleep.[92] Incorporation of tools measuring different facets of sleep disturbances are recommended.[91,92]

MANAGEMENT STRATEGIES

Management of patients with COFP and sleep disorders should be tailored to individualized needs. It is essential to treat any comorbid medical conditions, psychiatric illnesses, and/or substance abuse that may be precipitating or exacerbating their pain and/or their sleep disorders and to refer each patient to the relevant medical discipline according to the precipitating illness. An algorithm for management of patients with sleep disorders and COFP is presented in **Fig. 3**.

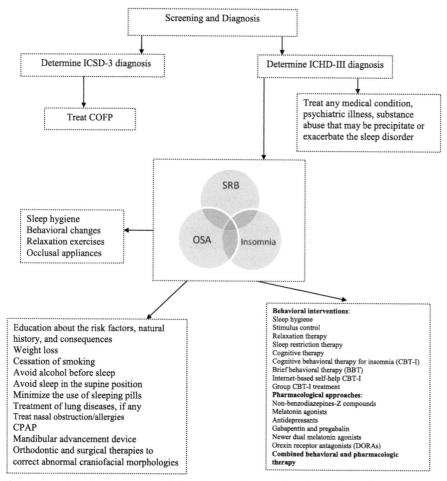

Fig. 3. Algorithm for management of patients with sleep disorders and orofacial pain. BBT, brief behavioral therapy; CBT-I, cognitive behavior therapy for insomnia; CPAP, continuous positive airway pressure; DORAs, dual orexin receptor antagonists; ICHD-II, International Classification of Headache Disorders, 3rd edition. (*Adapted from* Almoznino G, Benoliel R, Sharav Y, et al. Sleep disorders and chronic craniofacial pain: characteristics and management possibilities. Sleep Med Rev 2017;33:44; with permission.)

If screening and assessment by the dentist (see **Figs. 1** and **2**) reveals COFP and comorbid sleep disorders, such as insomnia, the patient should be referred to specialists as needed. COFP may be managed by an orofacial pain practitioner and sleep disorders should be managed by a sleep medicine specialist.[7] A multidisciplinary approach to the management of sleep disorders in patients with COFP should follow based on a biopsychosocial model of health.[7] Brousseau and colleagues[93] suggested a 4-step management algorithm for the assessment and treatment of sleep problems in patients with chronic pain: (1) evaluation for primary sleep disorder; (2) review of sleep hygiene; (3) behavioral and cognitive strategies; and (4) pharmacologic interventions.

An abortive or prophylactic individualized management approach, tailored to the COFP and sleep disorders, should be adopted. Discussion of specific medications used for the management of COFP and a comprehensive management approach can be found elsewhere.[7] However, the effects of COFP treatments on sleep should be taken into account to avoid aggravating preexisting sleep complaints or to potentiate the sleep effects of the medications in a beneficial manner.[94]

Treatment of the underlying sleep disorders (SRB, OSA, and restless legs syndrome) can greatly reduce pains such as headaches.[95] Considering that there is often an overlap between sleep disorders (see **Fig. 3**), a combination of treatment modalities should be used.

Management of Obstructive Sleep Apnea in Patients with Chronic Orofacial Pain

Management includes behavior modifications, such as weight loss; exercising; avoidance of smoking, alcohol, and certain medications (eg, sedatives, narcotics, and muscle relaxants); sleeping in a nonsupine position (if OSA is positional); and treatment of related medical conditions.

Continuous positive airway pressure (CPAP) is indicated as an initial therapy. Nonadherent patients with mild or moderate OSA may use mandibular advancement appliances (MAAs) during sleep. CPAP or bilevel positive airway pressure devices may improve or resolve headaches or may increase headache frequency, highlighting the need for individualizing patient care.

Orthodontic and surgical therapies to correct abnormal craniofacial morphologies can be considered.[95] However, there is insufficient evidence to recommend the use of drug therapy in the treatment of OSA.[96]

Management of Sleep-Related Bruxism in Patients with Chronic Orofacial Pain

Currently there is no cure for SRB and management consists of sleep hygiene, behavioral strategies, pharmacotherapy, and oral appliance therapy (OAT), although these management strategies are not yet fully evidence based.[90] The mechanism of action for OAT remains elusive while there is no evidence to support its role in stopping SRB[90,95] or TMD.[97] Furthermore, the initial decrease in the rhythmic masticatory muscle activity index in the first period of treatment seems to be transitory, and values return to baseline after a short time.[90] Paradoxically, some patients with SRB display increased EMG activity during sleep when wearing an OAT device.[90]

When SRB is related to OSA, using CPAP may eliminate SRB.[98] MAAs have been also shown to reduce SRB and may be considered for patients with SRB with concomitant OSA.[90]

Management of Insomnia in Patients with Chronic Orofacial Pain

The 2 most widely accepted treatment options for insomnia are cognitive behavior therapy (CBT) for insomnia (CBT-I) and hypnotic medications.[99–101] There has also been an increasing body of literature supporting the benefits of integrative medicine for patients with insomnia. Mind-body interventions such as hypnotherapy, meditation, guided imagery, mindfulness-based stress reduction, biofeedback, yoga, traditional Chinese practices (eg, qi gong, tai chi), and music therapy represent safe and cost-effective treatment options for insomnia and other sleep quality disturbances.[100,102,103]

Nonpharmacologic

Behavioral modalities for insomnia include sleep hygiene, CBT-I, multicomponent behavioral therapy or brief behavioral therapy (BBT) for insomnia, and other interventions, such as stimulus control, relaxation strategies, and sleep restriction.[100,101,104]

Management of insomnia should begin with nonpharmacologic treatment,[100,104] because of potential side effects, drug interactions, and risk of substance abuse associated with pharmacologic treatment.[100] Particularly, a nonpharmacologic approach is recommended in specific conditions, such as pregnancy and lactation; elderly patients; alcohol consumption; difficulties in swallowing pills; patients with kidney, liver, or lung disease; and in patients opposed to pharmacologic treatment.[99]

Furthermore, studies comparing medications with CBT-I showed similar short-term outcomes but improved long-term outcomes (up to 1 year) with CBT-I after treatment termination, suggesting a learned carry-over effect for CBT-I.[99,101] CBT interventions have also been used for pain, termed CBT for pain (CBT-P)[105]; however, studies that included sleep measures suggested minimal improvement in sleep after CBT-P.[106] Therefore, it was suggested that hybrid behavioral therapies, combining elements for both pain and sleep, be used to work synergistically on sleep and pain symptoms.[107,108] A meta-analysis of group CBT-I showed medium to large effect sizes for sleep onset latency, sleep efficiency, and wake after sleep onset and small effect sizes for pain outcomes.[109] CBT-I is effective in the treatment of insomnia secondary to chronic painful medical conditions such as fibromyalgia, mixed chronic pain conditions, back pain, arthritis, and osteoarthritis.[7] CBT-I strategies not only change sleep patterns but may also improve pain in adults, such as headaches[110] and TMD.[111]

Advantages and disadvantages of CBT-I and pharmacologic approaches to treat insomnia are presented in **Table 3**. Because of this, pharmacology is currently the primary treatment, whereas CBTI-I is used in only 1% of chronic insomniacs.[99,112] Lower cost and readily accessible options include bibliotherapy and telephone-based, Internet-based, or group CBT-I treatments.[100,101]

Pharmacologic

In contrast with CBT-I, which takes weeks, hypnotic medications act quickly, usually after the first dose, and are therefore preferred by many clinicians.[99] Approved US Food and Drug Administration (FDA) medications to treat insomnia include benzodiazepines, nonbenzodiazepine sedatives, the orexin receptor antagonist suvorexant, the melatonin receptor agonist ramelteon, and the antidepressant doxepin.[100,113,114]

The FDA recommends lower doses of hypnotics in women and in older or debilitated adults, as well as short-term use of these drugs (4–5 weeks), with the skills learned in CBT-I used to manage insomnia long term.[100] Further evaluation is recommended according to the FDA for patients with insomnia that does not resolve within 7 to 10 days of treatment.[100] However, none of the medications used to treat insomnia have been approved by any medical agency in the context of comorbid neurologic disease and they are therefore considered off-label. Moreover, the use of medication before the initiation of behavioral therapy seems to be less effective.[101] Because of risks of pharmacologic interventions (see **Table 3**), pharmacologic treatments are

Table 3
Advantages and disadvantages of cognitive behavioral therapy for insomnia and pharmacologic approaches to treat insomnia

	Advantages	Disadvantages

CBT-I	• Harms sparsely reported but likely small because of noninvasive nature of therapy
	• A learned carry-over effect
	• Better long-term outcomes
	• Suitable in specific conditions such as:
	  ○ Pregnancy and lactation
	  ○ Difficulties in swallowing pills
	  ○ Elderly
	  ○ Patients with kidney, liver, or lung disease
	  ○ Patients avoiding medications
		• Lack of insurance coverage
		• High initial cost
		• Few trained therapists
		• Treatment duration
		• Decreased effectiveness in older patients
		• Success related experience may be subjectively questionable
		• Sleep restriction may cause sleep deprivation therefore, if sleep time is significantly reduced, avoid hazardous activity and driving
		• Use with caution in bipolar disorder (sleep deprivation can trigger manic episodes)

Pharmacologic approaches	• Act quickly, usually after first dose • Usually covered by insurance • Lower initial cost	• Side effects • Drug interactions • Risk of substance abuse • Physical and psychological addiction with long-term use and withdrawal difficulties

Adapted from Almoznino G, Haviv Y, Sharav Y, et al. An update of management of insomnia in patients with chronic orofacial pain. Oral Dis 2017:23:1047; with permission.

recommended only when nonpharmacologic approaches fail or when insomnia persists after treatment of an underlying medical condition.[100,101] Another management approach includes combination therapy, in which CBT-I and a medication are initiated together (usually for 6 to 8 weeks), then the medication is tapered off or used per-demand while continuing CBT. However, combination therapy offers no short-term major advantage and only minimal long-term advantage.

The choice of the sedative-hypnotic is based on the insomnia type and the desirable effect duration: for sleep onset insomnia, short-acting medications (duration of effect ≤8 hours) are recommended; longer-acting medication is recommended in sleep maintenance insomnia, and zaleplon, as well as a sublingual tablet of zolpidem, is recommended for patients with awakening in the middle of the night, with the constraint that they are taken only if the patient has at least 4 hours in bed remaining.[101]

In COFP, a combination of pharmacologic therapies may be used as needed. For example, when the tricyclic antidepressant (TCA) often used in patients with COFP causes disturbed sleep, a benzodiazepine hypnotic or nonbenzodiazepine sedative may be used.

A summary of the FDA-approved medications to treat insomnia is presented in **Table 4**.

Benzodiazepines

There are 5 FDA-approved benzodiazepines for insomnia (estazolam, flurazepam, quazepam, temazepam, and triazolam).[99,100] Benzodiazepines are frequently used in patients with chronic pain and sleep disturbances. Benzodiazepines have been found

Table 4
US Food and Drug Administration–approved medications to treat insomnia

Pharmacologic Class	FDA-Approved Medications	Indications	Disadvantages
Benzodiazepines	Short acting • Triazolam Intermediate acting • Estazolam, • Temazepam Long acting • Flurazepam • Quazepam	• Insomnia • Sedative/hypnotic • Muscle relaxation • Anxiolysis • Pain relief • Anticonvulsant	• Daytime sedation, drowsiness, dizziness, or lightheadedness • Cognitive impairment and decreased attention • Rebound insomnia • Dependence and withdrawal difficulties • Respiratory suppression at high doses with coadministration of other drugs/substances (eg, alcohol) • Dementia • Increased risk for falls, hip fractures, and mobility problems in older adults • Temazepam associated with an increase in incident cancer cases
Nonbenzodiazepines: Z compounds	Short acting • Zolpidem • Zaleplon Long acting • Extended-release zolpidem • Eszopiclone	• As effective as benzodiazepines in insomnia treatment, but have fewer overall adverse effects • May reduce narcotic consumption • Middle-of-the-night awakenings	• FDA labels warn of daytime impairment, "sleep-driving," behavioral abnormalities, and worsening depression. Highest for extended-release and more prevalent in woman (eliminates slower than in men) and older adults • Observational studies have shown that hypnotic drugs may be associated with infrequent but serious adverse effects, such as dementia, serious injury, and fractures
Melatonin agonists	Ramelteon	• Circadian rhythm sleep disorder • Insomnia • Benzodiazepines withdrawal in elderly with insomnia • Preventive therapy in primary headaches • Analgesic effect	• Dizziness • Somnolence • Fatigue • Headache • Unpleasant taste • Nausea • New cognitive or behavioral abnormalities • Complex behaviors, such as sleep-driving • Exacerbation of depression and suicidal ideation in primarily depressed patients

(continued on next page)

Table 4
(continued)

Pharmacologic Class	FDA-Approved Medications	Indications	Disadvantages
Antidepressants	Doxepin	Doxepin: • Sleep maintenance insomnia Antidepressants: • Pain relief in COFP conditions • Preventive therapy in primary headaches • Useful in the management of patients with COFP with comorbid insomnia and depression	• Sedation • Fatigue • Weakness • Lethargy • Dry mouth and eyes • Constipation • Blurred vision • Headache • Orthostatic hypotension • Cardiac conduction delays • May prolong the QT interval
Orexin receptor antagonist	Suvorexant	• Sleep onset and sleep maintenance insomnia	• Because it is new to the market, fewer postmarket data are available and no trials have yet compared it with the other hypnotic drugs • Somnolence • Cognitive and behavioral changes, such as amnesia, anxiety, hallucinations, and other neuropsychiatric symptoms • Complex behaviors, such as sleep-driving; worsening of depression, including suicidal thinking in persons with depression • Daytime impairments • Sleep paralysis • Hypnagogic/ hypnopompic hallucinations

Adapted from Almoznino G, Haviv Y, Sharav Y, et al. An update of management of insomnia in patients with chronic orofacial pain. Oral Dis 2017:23:1048; with permission.

effective in treating pain in chronic tension headache, TMD, BMS, and TN.[115,116] In other studies, benzodiazepines failed to show a significant improvement in sleep in individuals with chronic pain conditions.[116]

Because of their potential side effects, benzodiazepines should be used at the lowest dose and for short periods (maximum 4 weeks), and daytime sedation, adverse effects, rebound insomnia, as well as dependence and withdrawal difficulties should be closely monitored. Careful medication selection to avoid dependence and respiratory suppression is critical in patients with pain, because of frequent coadministration of opioids, antiepileptic agents, neuropathic agents, and muscle relaxants.

Nonbenzodiazepine hypnotics

The nonbenzodiazepine Z compounds are as effective as benzodiazepines with fewer overall adverse effects. Nonbenzodiazepine hypnotics approved by the FDA for the treatment of insomnia include zolpidem, zolpidem extended-release, zaleplon, and eszopiclone.[100]

Interestingly, occasional side effects of these drugs include headaches. Zolpidem and eszopiclone improved sleep and quality of life in patients with fibromyalgia and rheumatoid arthritis.[117] However, although zolpidem, but not zopiclone, improved some sleep parameters in patients with fibromyalgia, neither drug improved pain.[118]

Melatonin

Melatonin is not FDA approved and is available over the counter; however, ramelteon, a melatonin receptor agonist, was approved by the FDA for the treatment of sleep onset insomnia. Melatonin is usually well tolerated, with few adverse effects, and therefore seems to be safe for short-term use (3 months or less).[100] Melatonin was found to be effective for preventive therapy in primary headaches and migraines,[119] in particular in CH, in which melatonin treatment is thought to reset the circadian pacemaker.[119] A positive response to melatonin was reported on hemicrania continua, fibromyalgia, and irritable bowel syndrome.[120] Melatonin lowered pain scores and reduced analgesic consumption in patients with TMD.[121] Furthermore, the effect of melatonin on pain seems to be independent of changes in sleep quality.[121]

Antidepressants

The TCAs are the main class of antidepressants used in headache treatment, with amitriptyline being the most studied. Antidepressants can also cause sedation by blocking acetylcholine, histamine, norepinephrine, and 5-HT. However, antidepressants are not all equal in improving sleep,[12,122] whereby some have been shown to improve sleep (amitriptyline, nortriptyline, trimipramine, and doxepin)[12,122] and others disturb sleep (desipramine and imipramine).[123] Sedating effect tends to be short-lived and other side effects are common, and the routine use of TCAs other than doxepin to treat insomnia in nondepressed patients has not been recommended.[94] Moreover, data on the use of antidepressants in the management of sleep in patients with pain disorders are limited.

Gabapentin and pregabalin

These anticonvulsant agents are commonly used in COFP conditions and also to manage patients with comorbid insomnia and chronic pain.[7] A systematic review concluded that pregabalin is beneficial in the treatment of sleep disturbances and pain symptoms in patients with fibromyalgia.[124] Significant reductions in pain and pain-related sleep interference were observed when pregabalin was used in the treatment of neuropathic pain.[125]

Orexin receptor antagonist

Antagonists that reversibly block the action of endogenous peptides at both the OX-1 and OX-2 receptors are termed dual orexin receptor antagonists (DORAs) and work by inhibiting the activation of the arousal system.[101] Suvorexant is a reversible DORA that was FDA approved for use for insomnia in 2014.[100,101] It is effective in treatment of sleep onset and sleep maintenance insomnia; however, no trials have yet compared it with the other hypnotic drugs.[101]

SUMMARY

The relationship between sleep disturbances and COFP represents a major challenge in clinical practice, particularly in the area of management. Sometimes, especially in refractory cases, despite the best intentions of the practitioner, management of orofacial pain is less than satisfactory, so a modification of diagnostic approaches may be needed, with greater focus on the identification of possible comorbidities, including sleep disturbances. This requirement implies the urgent need for a multidisciplinary and integrated approach to manage these patients with these comorbidities so as to increase the chances of pain relief and interventional success.

REFERENCES

1. Haack M, Mullington JM. Sustained sleep restriction reduces emotional and physical well-being. Pain 2005;119(1–3):56–64.
2. Haack M, Sanchez E, Mullington JM. Elevated inflammatory markers in response to prolonged sleep restriction are associated with increased pain experience in healthy volunteers. Sleep 2007;30(9):1145–52.
3. Lavigne GJ, Nashed A, Manzini C, et al. Does sleep differ among patients with common musculoskeletal pain disorders? Curr Rheumatol Rep 2011;13(6): 535–42.
4. American Academy of Sleep Medicine. International classification of sleep disorders. Darien (CT): American Academy of Sleep Medicine; 2014.
5. Merskey H, Bogduk N. Descriptions of chronic pain syndromes and definitions of pain terms. Classification of chronic pain. 2nd edition. Seattle (WA): IASP Press; 1994.
6. Williams AC, Craig KD. Updating the definition of pain. Pain 2016;157(11): 2420–3.
7. Sharav Y, Benoliel R. Orofacial pain and headache. 2nd edition. Chicago: Quintessence; 2015.
8. Linton SJ, MacDonald S. Pain and sleep disorders: clinical consequences and maintaining factors. In: Lavigne GS, Barry JS, Choiniere M, et al, editors. Sleep and pain. Seattle (WA): IASP Press; 2007. p. 417–37.
9. Institute of Medicine. Sleep disorders and sleep deprivation: an unmet public health problem. Washington, DC: The National Academies Press; 2006.
10. Centers for Disease Control and Prevention. Unhealthy sleep-related behaviors - 12 states, 2009. Morb Mortal Wkly Rep 2011;60:232–8.
11. Centers for Disease Control and Prevention. Effect of short sleep duration on daily activities—United States, 2005–2008. Morb Mortal Wkly Rep 2011;60: 239–42.
12. Cheatle MD, Foster S, Pinkett A, et al. Assessing and managing sleep disturbance in patients with chronic pain. Anesthesiol Clin 2016;34(2):379–93.
13. Benoliel R, Birman N, Eliav E, et al. The international classification of headache disorders: accurate diagnosis of orofacial pain? Cephalalgia 2008;28(7): 752–62.
14. Macfarlane TV, Worthington HV. Association between orofacial pain and other symptoms: a population-based study. Oral Biosci Med 2004;1:45–54.
15. Benoliel R, Eliav E, Sharav Y. Self-reports of pain-related awakenings in persistent orofacial pain patients. J Orofac Pain 2009;23(4):330–8.
16. Finan PH, Smith MT. The comorbidity of insomnia, chronic pain, and depression: dopamine as a putative mechanism. Sleep Med Rev 2013;17(3):173–83.

17. Bhaskar S, Hemavathy D, Prasad S. Prevalence of chronic insomnia in adult patients and its correlation with medical comorbidities. J Family Med Prim Care 2016;5(4):780–4.

18. Lavigne GJ, Sessle BJ. The neurobiology of orofacial pain and sleep and their interactions. J Dent Res 2016;95(10):1109–16.

19. Finan PH, Goodin BR, Smith MT. The association of sleep and pain: an update and a path forward. J Pain 2013;14(12):1539–52.

20. Melzack R. Pain and the neuromatrix in the brain. J Dent Educ 2001;65(12): 1378–82.

21. Barad MJ, Ueno T, Younger J, et al. Complex regional pain syndrome is associated with structural abnormalities in pain-related regions of the human brain. J Pain 2014;15(2):197–203.

22. Steiger A, Holsboer F. Neuropeptides and human sleep. Sleep 1997;20(11): 1038–52.

23. Riemann D, Voderholzer U, Spiegelhalder K, et al. Chronic insomnia and MRI-measured hippocampal volumes: a pilot study. Sleep 2007;30(8):955–8.

24. Spiegelhalder K, Regen W, Baglioni C, et al. Neuroimaging studies in insomnia. Curr Psychiatry Rep 2013;15(11):405.

25. Spiegelhalder K, Regen W, Baglioni C, et al. Insomnia does not appear to be associated with substantial structural brain changes. Sleep 2013;36(5):731–7.

26. Bjurstrom MF, Giron SE, Griffis CA. Cerebrospinal fluid cytokines and neurotrophic factors in human chronic pain populations: a comprehensive review. Pain Pract 2016;16(2):183–203.

27. Krueger JM, Rector DM, Churchill L. Sleep and cytokines. Sleep Med Clin 2007; 2(2):161–9.

28. Lautenbacher S, Kundermann B, Krieg JC. Sleep deprivation and pain perception. Sleep Med Rev 2006;10(5):357–69.

29. Russell IJ, Vaeroy H, Javors M, et al. Cerebrospinal fluid biogenic amine metabolites in fibromyalgia/fibrositis syndrome and rheumatoid arthritis. Arthritis Rheum 1992;35(5):550–6.

30. Kwon M, Altin M, Duenas H, et al. The role of descending inhibitory pathways on chronic pain modulation and clinical implications. Pain Pract 2014;14(7):656–67.

31. Mignot E, Taheri S, Nishino S. Sleeping with the hypothalamus: emerging therapeutic targets for sleep disorders. Nat Neurosci 2002;5(Suppl):1071–5.

32. Merrill RL. Orofacial pain and sleep. Sleep Med Clin 2010;5(1):131–44.

33. Sutcliffe JG, de Lecea L. The hypocretins: setting the arousal threshold. Nat Rev Neurosci 2002;3(5):339–49.

34. Ozcan M, Ayar A, Serhatlioglu I, et al. Orexins activates protein kinase C-mediated Ca(2+) signaling in isolated rat primary sensory neurons. Physiol Res 2010;59(2):255–62.

35. Holland P, Goadsby PJ. The hypothalamic orexinergic system: pain and primary headaches. Headache 2007;47(6):951–62.

36. Smith MT, Edwards RR, McCann UD, et al. The effects of sleep deprivation on pain inhibition and spontaneous pain in women. Sleep 2007;30(4):494–505.

37. Edwards RR, Grace E, Peterson S, et al. Sleep continuity and architecture: associations with pain-inhibitory processes in patients with temporomandibular joint disorder. Eur J Pain 2009;13(10):1043–7.

38. Bentley AJ, Newton S, Zio CD. Sensitivity of sleep stages to painful thermal stimuli. J Sleep Res 2003;12(2):143–7.

39. Lavigne G, Zucconi M, Castronovo C, et al. Sleep arousal response to experimental thermal stimulation during sleep in human subjects free of pain and sleep problems. Pain 2000;84(2–3):283–90.

40. Bastuji H, Perchet C, Legrain V, et al. Laser evoked responses to painful stimulation persist during sleep and predict subsequent arousals. Pain 2008;137(3): 589–99.

41. Moldofsky H. Sleep-wake mechanisms in fibrositis. J Rheumatol Suppl 1989;19: 47–8.

42. Almoznino G, Benoliel R, Sharav Y, et al. Sleep disorders and chronic craniofacial pain: Characteristics and management possibilities. Sleep Med Rev 2017; 33:39–50.

43. Kim J, Cho SJ, Kim WJ, et al. Insufficient sleep is prevalent among migraineurs: a population-based study. J Headache Pain 2017;18(1):50.

44. Kim J, Cho SJ, Kim WJ, et al. Insomnia in probable migraine: a population-based study. J Headache Pain 2016;17(1):92.

45. Yang CP, Wang SJ. Sleep in patients with chronic migraine. Curr Pain Headache Rep 2017;21(9):39.

46. Harnod T, Wang YC, Kao CH. Association of migraine and sleep-related breathing disorder: a population-based cohort study. Medicine (Baltimore) 2015; 94(36):e1506.

47. De Luca Canto G, Singh V, Bigal ME, et al. Association between tension-type headache and migraine with sleep bruxism: a systematic review. Headache 2014;54(9):1460–9.

48. Kristiansen HA, Kvaerner KJ, Akre H, et al. Migraine and sleep apnea in the general population. J Headache Pain 2011;12(1):55–61.

49. Freedom T. Headaches and sleep disorders. Dis Mon 2015;61(6):240–8.

50. Kim J, Cho SJ, Kim WJ, et al. Insomnia in tension-type headache: a population-based study. J Headache Pain 2017;18(1):95.

51. Chiu YC, Hu HY, Lee FP, et al. Tension-type headache associated with obstructive sleep apnea: a nationwide population-based study. J Headache Pain 2015; 16:34.

52. Kristiansen HA, Kvaerner KJ, Akre H, et al. Tension-type headache and sleep apnea in the general population. J Headache Pain 2011;12(1):63–9.

53. Barloese MC. Neurobiology and sleep disorders in cluster headache. J Headache Pain 2015;16:562.

54. Evers S, Barth B, Frese A, et al. Sleep apnea in patients with cluster headache: a case-control study. Cephalalgia 2014;34(10):828–32.

55. Pfaffenrath V, Pollmann W, Ruther E, et al. Onset of nocturnal attacks of chronic cluster headache in relation to sleep stages. Acta Neurol Scand 1986;73(4): 403–7.

56. Terzaghi M, Ghiotto N, Sances G, et al. Episodic cluster headache: NREM prevalence of nocturnal attacks. Time to look beyond macrostructural analysis? Headache 2010;50(6):1050–4.

57. Devor M, Wood I, Sharav Y, et al. Trigeminal neuralgia during sleep. Pain Pract 2008;8(4):263–8.

58. Haviv Y, Zini A, Etzioni Y, et al. The impact of chronic orofacial pain on daily life: the vulnerable patient and disruptive pain. Oral Surg Oral Med Oral Pathol Oral Radiol 2017;123(1):58–66.

59. Lee DH, Park JE, Yoon DM, et al. Factors associated with increased risk for clinical insomnia in patients with postherpetic neuralgia: a retrospective cross-sectional study. Pain Med 2016;17(10):1917–22.

60. Mehta N, Bucior I, Bujanover S, et al. Relationship between pain relief, reduction in pain-associated sleep interference, and overall impression of improvement in patients with postherpetic neuralgia treated with extended-release gabapentin. Health Qual Life Outcomes 2016;14:54.

61. Chainani-Wu N, Madden E, Silverman S Jr. A case-control study of burning mouth syndrome and sleep dysfunction. Oral Surg Oral Med Oral Pathol Oral Radiol Endod 2011;112(2):203–8.

62. Lopez-Jornet P, Lucero-Berdugo M, Castillo-Felipe C, et al. Assessment of self-reported sleep disturbance and psychological status in patients with burning mouth syndrome. J Eur Acad Dermatol Venereol 2015;29(7):1285–90.

63. Adamo D, Schiavone V, Aria M, et al. Sleep disturbance in patients with burning mouth syndrome: a case-control study. J Orofac Pain 2013;27(4):304–13.

64. Adamo D, Sardella A, Varoni E, et al. The association between burning mouth syndrome and sleep disturbance: a case-control multicentre study. Oral Dis 2018;24(4):638–49.

65. Lee CF, Lin KY, Lin MC, et al. Sleep disorders increase the risk of burning mouth syndrome: a retrospective population-based cohort study. Sleep Med 2014; 15(11):1405–10.

66. Benoliel R, Zini A, Zakuto A, et al. Subjective sleep quality in temporomandibular disorder patients and association with disease characteristics and oral health-related quality of life. J Oral Facial Pain Headache 2017;31(4):313–22.

67. Vazquez-Delgado E, Schmidt JE, Carlson CR, et al. Psychological and sleep quality differences between chronic daily headache and temporomandibular disorders patients. Cephalalgia 2004;24(6):446–54.

68. Collesano V, Segu M, Masseroli C, et al. Temporomandibular disorders and sleep disorders: which relationship? Minerva Stomatol 2004;53(11–12):661–8.

69. Sanders AE, Akinkugbe AA, Bair E, et al. Subjective sleep quality deteriorates before development of painful temporomandibular disorder. J Pain 2016; 17(6):669–77.

70. Dubrovsky B, Janal MN, Lavigne GJ, et al. Depressive symptoms account for differences between self-reported versus polysomnographic assessment of sleep quality in women with myofascial TMD. J Oral Rehabil 2017;44(12): 925–33.

71. Geng W, Wu G, Huang F, et al. Sleep deprivation induces abnormal bone metabolism in temporomandibular joint. Int J Clin Exp Med 2015;8(1):395–403.

72. Ma C, Wu G, Wang Z, et al. Effects of chronic sleep deprivation on the extracellular signal-regulated kinase pathway in the temporomandibular joint of rats. PLoS One 2014;9(9):e107544.

73. Wu G, Chen L, Wei G, et al. Effects of sleep deprivation on pain-related factors in the temporomandibular joint. J Surg Res 2014;192(1):103–11.

74. Kou XX, Wu YW, Ding Y, et al. 17beta-estradiol aggravates temporomandibular joint inflammation through the NF-kappaB pathway in ovariectomized rats. Arthritis Rheum 2011;63(7):1888–97.

75. Dias GM, Bonato LL, Guimaraes JP, et al. A study of the association between sleep bruxism, low quality of sleep, and degenerative changes of the temporomandibular joint. J Craniofac Surg 2015;26(8):2347–50.

76. Cao R, Huang F, Wang P, et al. Chronic sleep deprivation alters the myosin heavy chain isoforms in the masseter muscle in rats. Br J Oral Maxillofac Surg 2015;53(5):430–5.

77. Yujra VQ, Antunes HKM, Monico-Neto M, et al. Sleep deprivation induces pathological changes in rat masticatory muscles: role of toll like signaling pathway and atrophy. J Cell Biochem 2018;119(2):2269–77.

78. Lei J, Liu MQ, Yap AU, et al. Sleep disturbance and psychologic distress: prevalence and risk indicators for temporomandibular disorders in a Chinese population. J Oral Facial Pain Headache 2015;29(1):24–30.

79. Lin WC, Shen CC, Tsai SJ, et al. Increased risk of myofascial pain syndrome among patients with insomnia. Pain Med 2017;18(8):1557–65.

80. Dubrovsky B, Raphael KG, Lavigne GJ, et al. Polysomnographic investigation of sleep and respiratory parameters in women with temporomandibular pain disorders. J Clin Sleep Med 2014;10(2):195–201.

81. Schmitter M, Kares-Vrincianu A, Kares H, et al. Sleep-associated aspects of myofascial pain in the orofacial area among temporomandibular disorder patients and controls. Sleep Med 2015;16(9):1056–61.

82. Reissmann DR, John MT, Aigner A, et al. Interaction between awake and sleep bruxism is associated with increased presence of painful temporomandibular disorder. J Oral Facial Pain Headache 2017;31(4):299–305.

83. Muzalev K, Lobbezoo F, Janal MN, et al. Interepisode sleep bruxism intervals and myofascial face pain. Sleep 2017;40(8). https://doi.org/10.1093/sleep/zsx078.

84. Raphael KG, Sirois DA, Janal MN, et al. Sleep bruxism and myofascial temporomandibular disorders: a laboratory-based polysomnographic investigation. J Am Dent Assoc 2012;143(11):1223–31.

85. Jimenez-Silva A, Pena-Duran C, Tobar-Reyes J, et al. Sleep and awake bruxism in adults and its relationship with temporomandibular disorders: a systematic review from 2003 to 2014. Acta Odontol Scand 2017;75(1):36–58.

86. Budhiraja R, Roth T, Hudgel DW, et al. Prevalence and polysomnographic correlates of insomnia comorbid with medical disorders. Sleep 2011;34(7):859–67.

87. Medarov BI, Victorson DE, Judson MA. Patient-reported outcome measures for sleep disorders and related problems: clinical and research applications. Chest 2013;143(6):1809–18.

88. Ramakrishnan K, Scheid DC. Treatment options for insomnia. Am Fam Physician 2007;76(4):517–26.

89. Qaseem A, Dallas P, Owens DK, et al. Diagnosis of obstructive sleep apnea in adults: a clinical practice guideline from the American College of Physicians. Ann Intern Med 2014;161(3):210–20.

90. Carra MC, Huynh N, Fleury B, et al. Overview on sleep bruxism for sleep medicine clinicians. Sleep Med Clin 2015;10(3):375–84, xvi.

91. Klingman KJ, Jungquist CR, Perlis ML. Questionnaires that screen for multiple sleep disorders. Sleep Med Rev 2017;32:37–44.

92. Sommer I, Lavigne G, Ettlin DA. Review of self-reported instruments that measure sleep dysfunction in patients suffering from temporomandibular disorders and/or orofacial pain. Sleep Med 2015;16(1):27–38.

93. Brousseau M, Manzini C, Thie N, et al. Understanding and managing the interaction between sleep and pain: an update for the dentist. J Can Dent Assoc 2003;69(7):437–42.

94. Nesbitt AD, Leschziner GD, Peatfield RC. Headache, drugs and sleep. Cephalalgia 2014;34(10):756–66.

95. Carra MC, Bruni O, Huynh N. Topical review: sleep bruxism, headaches, and sleep-disordered breathing in children and adolescents. J Orofac Pain 2012;26(4):267–76.

96. Mason M, Welsh EJ, Smith I. Drug therapy for obstructive sleep apnoea in adults. Cochrane Database Syst Rev 2013;(5):CD003002.

97. Katyayan PA, Katyayan MK, Shah RJ, et al. Efficacy of appliance therapy on temporomandibular disorder related facial pain and mandibular mobility: a randomized controlled study. J Indian Prosthodont Soc 2014;14(3):251–61.

98. Oksenberg A, Arons E. Sleep bruxism related to obstructive sleep apnea: the effect of continuous positive airway pressure. Sleep Med 2002;3(6):513–5.

99. Asnis GM, Thomas M, Henderson MA. Pharmacotherapy treatment options for insomnia: a primer for clinicians. Int J Mol Sci 2015;17(1). pii:E50.

100. Qaseem A, Kansagara D, Forciea MA, et al. Management of chronic insomnia disorder in adults: a clinical practice guideline from the American College of Physicians. Ann Intern Med 2016;165(2):125–33.

101. Kay-Stacey M, Attarian H. Advances in the management of chronic insomnia. BMJ 2016;354:i2123.

102. Kligler B, Teets R, Quick M. Complementary/integrative therapies that work: a review of the evidence. Am Fam Physician 2016;94(5):369–74.

103. Lin YF, Liu ZD, Ma W, et al. Hazards of insomnia and the effects of acupuncture treatment on insomnia. J Integr Med 2016;14(3):174–86.

104. Brasure M, Fuchs E, MacDonald R, et al. Psychological and behavioral interventions for managing insomnia disorder: an evidence report for a clinical practice guideline by the American College of Physicians. Ann Intern Med 2016;165(2): 113–24.

105. Glombiewski JA, Hartwich-Tersek J, Rief W. Two psychological interventions are effective in severely disabled, chronic back pain patients: a randomised controlled trial. Int J Behav Med 2010;17(2):97–107.

106. Tang NK. Cognitive-behavioral therapy for sleep abnormalities of chronic pain patients. Curr Rheumatol Rep 2009;11(6):451–60.

107. Finan PH, Buenaver LF, Coryell VT, et al. Cognitive-behavioral therapy for comorbid insomnia and chronic pain. Sleep Med Clin 2014;9(2):261–74.

108. Tang NK, Goodchild CE, Salkovskis PM. Hybrid cognitive-behaviour therapy for individuals with insomnia and chronic pain: a pilot randomised controlled trial. Behav Res Ther 2012;50(12):814–21.

109. Koffel EA, Koffel JB, Gehrman PR. A meta-analysis of group cognitive behavioral therapy for insomnia. Sleep Med Rev 2015;19:6–16.

110. Lipchik GL, Nash JM. Cognitive-behavioral issues in the treatment and management of chronic daily headache. Curr Pain Headache Rep 2002;6(6):473–9.

111. Ferrando M, Galdon MJ, Dura E, et al. Enhancing the efficacy of treatment for temporomandibular patients with muscular diagnosis through cognitive-behavioral intervention, including hypnosis: a randomized study. Oral Surg Oral Med Oral Pathol Oral Radiol 2012;113(1):81–9.

112. Riemann D, Spiegelhalder K, Espie C, et al. Chronic insomnia: clinical and research challenges–an agenda. Pharmacopsychiatry 2011;44(1):1–14.

113. Wilt TJ, MacDonald R, Brasure M, et al. Pharmacologic treatment of insomnia disorder: an evidence report for a clinical practice guideline by the American College of Physicians. Ann Intern Med 2016;165(2):103–12.

114. Sateia MJ, Buysse DJ, Krystal AD, et al. Clinical practice guideline for the pharmacologic treatment of chronic insomnia in adults: an American Academy of Sleep Medicine Clinical Practice Guideline. J Clin Sleep Med 2017;13(2): 307–49.

115. Spanemberg JC, Rodriguez de Rivera Campillo E, Salas EJ, et al. Burning mouth syndrome: update. Oral Health Dent Manag 2014;13(2):418–24.

116. Nielsen S, Lintzeris N, Bruno R, et al. Benzodiazepine use among chronic pain patients prescribed opioids: associations with pain, physical and mental health, and health service utilization. Pain Med 2015;16(2):356–66.

117. Roth T, Price JM, Amato DA, et al. The effect of eszopiclone in patients with insomnia and coexisting rheumatoid arthritis: a pilot study. Prim Care Companion J Clin Psychiatry 2009;11(6):292–301.

118. Roehrs TA. Does effective management of sleep disorders improve pain symptoms? Drugs 2009;69(Suppl 2):5–11.

119. Bougea A, Spantideas N, Lyras V, et al. Melatonin 4 mg as prophylactic therapy for primary headaches: a pilot study. Funct Neurol 2016;31(1):33–7.

120. Rozen TD. How effective is melatonin as a preventive treatment for hemicrania continua? A clinic-based study. Headache 2015;55(3):430–6.

121. Vidor LP, Torres IL, Custodio de Souza IC, et al. Analgesic and sedative effects of melatonin in temporomandibular disorders: a double-blind, randomized, parallel-group, placebo-controlled study. J Pain Symptom Manage 2013;46(3): 422–32.

122. Mayers AG, Baldwin DS. Antidepressants and their effect on sleep. Hum Psychopharmacol 2005;20(8):533–59.

123. Sonntag A, Rothe B, Guldner J, et al. Trimipramine and imipramine exert different effects on the sleep EEG and on nocturnal hormone secretion during treatment of major depression. Depression 1996;4(1):1–13.

124. Straube S, Derry S, Moore RA, et al. Pregabalin in fibromyalgia–responder analysis from individual patient data. BMC Musculoskelet Disord 2010;11:150.

125. Anastassiou E, Iatrou CA, Vlaikidis N, et al. Impact of pregabalin treatment on pain, pain-related sleep interference and general well-being in patients with neuropathic pain: a non-interventional, multicentre, post-marketing study. Clin Drug Investig 2011;31(6):417–26.

Sleep Bruxism and Pain

Eduardo E. Castrillon, DDS, MSc, PhD[a,b,*],
Fernando G. Exposto, DDS, MSc[a,b]

KEYWORDS

- Sleep bruxism • Orofacial pain • Headache

KEY POINTS

- In clinical practice it is common to base conclusions and treatments plans on paradigms supported by evidence that suggests that many different harmful oral health outcomes are reported to be associated with bruxism such as tooth wear, masticatory muscle tenderness, headaches and painful TMD.
- The association between TMD, headaches and bruxism has been discussed and argued for many years. Despite this with the available scientific evidence it is doubtful that bruxism is a direct cause of pain and therefore treatments strategies focused on controlling bruxism in order to decrease pain may not be the best solution for patients showing both conditions.

INTRODUCTION

Grinding the teeth has been described as an oral behavior that humans engage in related to the perception of pain and anger; it is even reported in the Old Testament of the Bible. This oral behavior was later defined as "bruxism" and this word has its origins in the Greek word *brygmos* (βρυγμός) that means gnashing of the teeth.[1] This behavior was scientifically described for the first time in the early 1900s.[2]

Today bruxism may be defined as "a repetitive jaw-muscle activity characterized by clenching or grinding of the teeth and/or by bracing or thrusting of the mandible."[3] Bruxism has 2 distinct circadian manifestations: it can occur during sleep (indicated as sleep bruxism [SB]) or during wakefulness (indicated as awake bruxism [AB]).[3] These 2 distinct manifestations of bruxism may not be just 2 manifestations of the same entity that occurs in different circadian phases (sleep or awake) but more likely are 2 distinct entities that, even though they may share common risk factors and lead to similar consequences on the masticatory system, may have different etiology and pathophysiology.[4] Moreover, it has been proposed that bruxism should be diagnosed using a grading system that categorizes the diagnoses based on the methods used

Disclosure: The authors have nothing to disclose.
[a] Section of Orofacial Pain and Jaw Function, Department of Dentistry and Oral Health, Aarhus University, Aarhus, Denmark; [b] Scandinavian Center for Orofacial Neurosciences (SCON)
* Corresponding author. Vennelyst Boulevard 9, Aarhus 8000, Denmark.
E-mail address: EC@dent.au.dk

into possible (self-report and questionnaires), probable (clinical signs and symptoms), and definitive (polysomnography) bruxism.[3]

The scientific knowledge in the field of bruxism has increased largely in recent years with more information being obtained about SB than AB. Despite the progress achieved in the knowledge of bruxism, many questions remain unanswered. With this available knowledge it has been suggested that bruxism can only be defined as an "oral behavior that may lead to harm" and it cannot be labeled as a harmful dysfunction itself (ie, disorder) or even a risk factor for harmful oral health outcomes.[5] Moreover, the scientific evidence has indicated that the focus of bruxism etiology should be changed from peripheral to central mechanisms[6] and occlusion can be categorically disregarded as an etiology of bruxism.[7]

In clinical practice, it is common to base conclusions and treatments plans on paradigms supported by evidence that suggests that many different harmful oral health outcomes are reported to be associated with bruxism, such as tooth wear, masticatory muscle tenderness, headaches, and painful temporomandibular disorders (TMDs).[8–10] This evidence leads to a simplistic cause-effect model based on the assumption that bruxism causes pain due to an overload of the masticatory system and also that higher bruxism muscle activity leads to more pain.[11] This article critically examines the current evidence that links pain (TMD and headache) and SB.

BRUXISM AND PAIN: COMPLICATIONS IN DRAWING CONNECTIONS

The challenge in accepting a simplistic cause-effect model is that a large part of the available scientific information is based mainly on studies where self-report (possible bruxism) is the diagnostic method used.[9,12] At this time, the reliability of the self-report method to determine the real existence of SB has been demonstrated as low,[13] with a reported sensitivity of 50% and specificity of 73%.[4] Nevertheless, it is still one of the most used methods (clinically and for research) to diagnose bruxism due to difficult access to gold standard diagnostic methods (polysomnography) that can aid in establishing a definitive bruxism diagnosis (sensitivity of 74% and specificity of 90%).[4] Despite all the limitations of the self-report method, patients suffering from TMDs often self-report (probable bruxism) more bruxism activity than non-TMD patients.[14] This difference disappears when a diagnosis of SB is confirmed by means of polysomnography (definitive bruxism).[15] As discussed previously, it is currently accepted that bruxism has 2 distinct circadian manifestations—SB and AB[3]—that may have different etiology and pathophysiology,[4] therefore making it difficult to validate and interpret the results of studies in which this variable was not taken into account, as evidenced by a published systematic review of headaches and bruxism.[16]

Another complication in interpreting the relationship between bruxism and orofacial pain is that changes in classifications of TMDs[17,18] and headaches[19] make recent results difficult to compare with findings reported using earlier classifications. For example, in cases of a diagnosis of "headache attributed to TMD" or tension-type headache (TTH), it is not clear if a reported headache could actually be myalgia of the temporalis muscle and as such should not be given a headache diagnosis but a TMD diagnosis. Furthermore, most of the studies looking at the association between bruxism and headache do not take into account the diagnosis of medication-overuse headache that may cause morning headaches and, according to the literature, makes up 25% to 50% of the chronic headache population.[20]

Additionally, there are studies that suggest that bruxism may lead to the development of headaches[8] and also to the development of TMDs.[12,21] This makes the relationship and limits between bruxism/headache and bruxism/TMD difficult to understand due to their overlap. Furthermore, obstructive sleep apnea (OSA) has been associated with SB[22] and also may be related to TMD[23]; approximately 50% of OSA patients have headache.[24] Taking all this evidence together complicates even more the understanding of the relationship between painful TMD, headache, and SB.

MYOFASCIAL PAIN AND SLEEP BRUXISM

Bruxism is an oral behavior characterized by increased repetitive jaw-muscle activity[3] "that may lead to harm"[5] the facial muscle tissue and may be perceived as pain, such as in painful muscular TMD.[25] As suggested previously, there are several complications in establishing a direct connection between bruxism and pain. The simplistic cause-effect view is based on the assumption that bruxism causes pain due to an overloaded masticatory system and this effect may be dose-responsive (for example, higher bruxism muscle activity leads to more pain). In accordance with this view, it is logical to demonstrate this assumption by manipulating or assessing the electromyographic (EMG) activity to see if it has a direct effect over pain perception. This view has been challenged by several studies that demonstrated that sleep bruxers who show no painful symptoms have higher EMG activity than those with painful symptoms,[26] and EMG activity in patients with painful TMDs did not showed higher EMG activity than healthy controls.[27] Moreover, bruxers with low frequency of EMG activity have been shown to report craniofacial pain more frequently.[28] This apparent contradiction may be explained by the pain-adaptation model proposed by Lund and colleagues.[29] Conversely, when high-frequency EMG activity patients who report muscle pain have their EMG manipulated and subsequently decreased with contingent electrical stimulation, it does not reduce pain.[30]

Experiments manipulating the EMG activity of masticatory muscles suggest that, compared with healthy subjects, patients with TMDs become more easily fatigued, but the EMG activation process during the fatigue test is similar between healthy subjects and patients with TMDs.[31] Moreover, experimental bruxism studies with tooth clenching or tooth grinding in healthy human subjects have consistently shown low grades of painful symptoms, which quickly resolve, and no studies have so far been able to match the characteristics of delayed onset of muscle soreness seen in limb muscles. As such, it seems unlikely that transient or tissue injury–based pain alone can explain the clinical characteristics and manifestations of persistent craniofacial pain.[11] As suggested by Takeuchi and colleagues,[32] "tooth clenching alone is insufficient to initiate longer lasting and self-perpetuating symptoms of TMD, which may require other risk factors." Nevertheless, recent results published showed that this transient pain resulting from sustained elevated muscle activity (SEMA) is accompanied by changes in hemodynamics characteristics.[33] On the contrary, hemodynamics characteristics are not influenced by glutamate evoked pain after SEMA.[34] Additionally, experimentally evoked pain in the masseter muscle or TMJ did not show any robust effect in terms of bigger variability of bite force and jaw muscle activity during repeated splitting of food morsels.[35] Taking all this evidence together, it becomes difficult to establish a direct cause-effect relationship between bruxism and painful TMD diagnoses.

HEADACHES AND SLEEP BRUXISM

The International Classification of Headache Disorders (ICHD) establishes that headache could be a disease in itself (primary headaches) or a symptom of some other disease (secondary headaches).[19] In the group of primary headaches, TTH is the most common headache, affecting approximately 21% of the population, followed by migraine that affects approximately 15%.[36] It has been suggested that there is a relation between headaches (primary headaches, such as migraine and TTH) and TMDs.[37] Additionally, the recently added diagnosis of headache attributed to TMD shows comorbidity between headache and TMD[18,19] and this relationship may be mediated by, among other things, bruxism.[38]

The association between migraine and TTH with SB has been addressed recently in a published review that included only 2 studies that fulfilled the inclusion criteria of diagnosis of headaches according to the ICHD and the SB diagnosis according to the American Academy of Sleep Medicine,[16] evidencing that the relationship between SB and headache has been poorly studied.

The available evidence shows that the relationship between headache and SB seems confounded by TMD. This is because it has been showed that painful TMD, SB (especially self-report), and headaches are all significantly related.[9,12] On the other hand, it has been shown that SB alone does not increase the chances of suffering from any type of headache. Painful TMDs on the other hand significantly increased the risk for chronic and episodic migraine but not episodic TTH.[39] Moreover, a recent study found an association between migraine and TMDs but not between TTHs and TMDs and this relationship was confounded by the presence of bruxism.[38] This confirms a 3-way relationship between SB, headache, and TMD. Finally, in a study using a portable EMG device for 1 week, patients with TTH were not found to have more EMG activity per hour of sleep compared with healthy controls.[27] Furthermore, no difference was found between the EMG activity of TTH patients who self-reported SB compared with TTH patients who did not self-report SB,[27] demonstrating again the limitations interpreting the results due to limitations of self-reported SB.[13]

When assessing nonspecific headaches, it has been shown that the use of both a mandibular advancement device and a stabilization appliance can lead to a decrease in headache intensity and headache days by means of decreased rhythmic masticatory muscle activity.[40,41] In cases of mandibular advancement device,[40] it did not completely eliminate SB behavior but there was a decrease as assessed by decreased rhythmic masticatory muscle activity. On the other hand, 84% of patients reported a continuation of SB behavior after insertion of a stabilization appliance.[41] Taking these results together, the relationship between headaches and SB seems confounded by TMD.

Another complication in interpreting the scientific evidence available to determine relationships between headaches and bruxism is the responsibility for appropriately interpreting the report of morning headaches (affecting 5% of the general population)[42] that are not caused exclusively by SB.[43] Morning headaches may be due to primary headaches that have a circadian rhythm compatible with nocturnal or early morning headaches, such as migraine, cluster headache, and hypnic headache, OSA, medication-overuse headache, insomnia, and brain tumor.[44] Therefore, it is important for dentists to be aware of other possible causes of headache besides SB and importantly to identify if the morning headaches may be caused by a brain tumor. This can be identified if the morning headaches are accompanied by papilledema or vomiting and/or are made better by standing up; if s,o the patient should immediately be sent to an emergency department.

SUMMARY

The association between TMDs, headaches, and bruxism has been discussed and argued for many years. Despite this, pain continues to be one of the most discussed issues regarding the effects of bruxism.

The available scientific evidence is difficult to interpret due lack of scientific rigor in assessing bruxism and in the classification of TMDs and headaches. Nevertheless, pain (TMD/headache) is one of the common reports to coexist with self-reported bruxism.

In light of the available scientific evidence, it is doubtful that bruxism is a direct cause of pain and, therefore, treatments strategies focused on controlling bruxism to decrease pain may not be the best solution for patients showing both conditions. Clinicians should treat/manage both pain and bruxism at the same time and take into account that both problems have a multifactorial etiology.

Clinician efforts should be encouraged to acquire the minimum knowledge needed to evaluate and identify the relationships/coexistence of patients with sign and symptoms of bruxism, TMD, headache, and/or OSA.

Further research is needed into this association (bruxism, TMD, headache, and/or OSA) with higher methodological rigor.

REFERENCES

1. Svensson P, Arima T, Lavigne GJ, et al. Sleep bruxism. In: Kryger M, Roth T, Dement WC, editors. Principles and practice of sleep medicine. 6th edition. Elsevier; 2017. p. 1423–6, e1424.
2. Marie MM, Pietkiewicz M. La bruxomanie. Rev Stomatol 1907;107.
3. Lobbezoo F, Ahlberg J, Glaros AG, et al. Bruxism defined and graded: an international consensus. J Oral Rehabil 2013;40(1):2–4.
4. Carra MC. Sleep-related bruxism. Curr Sleep Med Rep 2018;4(1):28–38.
5. Raphael KG, Santiago V, Lobbezoo F. Is bruxism a disorder or a behaviour? Rethinking the international consensus on defining and grading of bruxism. J Oral Rehabil 2016;43(10):791–8.
6. Lobbezoo F, Naeije M. Bruxism is mainly regulated centrally, not peripherally. J Oral Rehabil 2001;28(12):1085–91.
7. Lobbezoo F, Ahlberg J, Manfredini D, et al. Are bruxism and the bite causally related? J Oral Rehabil 2012;39(7):489–501.
8. Villarosa GA, Moss RA. Oral behavioral patterns as factors contributing to the development of head and facial pain. J Prosthet Dent 1985;54(3):427–30.
9. Huang GJ, LeResche L, Critchlow CW, et al. Risk factors for diagnostic subgroups of painful Temporomandibular Disorders (TMD). J Dent Res 2002;81(4):284–8.
10. Camparis CM, Siqueira JTT. Sleep bruxism: clinical aspects and characteristics in patients with and without chronic orofacial pain. Oral Surg Oral Med Oral Pathol Oral Radiol Endod 2006;101(2):188–93.
11. Svensson P, Jadidi F, Arima T, et al. Relationships between craniofacial pain and bruxism. J Oral Rehabil 2008;35(7):524–47.
12. Ohrbach R, Bair E, Fillingim RB, et al. Clinical orofacial characteristics associated with risk of first-onset TMD: the OPPERA prospective cohort study. J Pain 2013; 14(12 Suppl):T33–50.
13. Maluly M, Andersen ML, Dal-Fabbro C, et al. Polysomnographic study of the prevalence of sleep bruxism in a population sample. J Dent Res 2013;92(7 Suppl):S97–103, 35(7):524–47.
14. Manfredini D, Lobbezoo F. Relationship between bruxism and temporomandibular disorders: a systematic review of literature from 1998 to 2008. Oral Surg Oral Med Oral Pathol Oral Radiol Endod 2010;109(6):e26–50.

15. Raphael KG, Sirois DA, Janal MN, et al. Sleep bruxism and myofascial temporo-mandibular disorders: a laboratory-based polysomnographic investigation. J Am Dent Assoc 2012;143(11):1223–31.

16. De Luca Canto G, Singh V, Bigal ME, et al. Association between tension-type headache and migraine with sleep bruxism: a systematic review. Headache 2014;54(9):1460–9.

17. Schiffman E, Ohrbach R, List T, et al. Diagnostic criteria for headache attributed to temporomandibular disorders. Cephalalgia 2012;32(9):683–92.

18. Schiffman E, Ohrbach R, Truelove E, et al. Diagnostic criteria for temporomandibular disorders (DC/TMD) for clinical and research applications: recommendations of the international RDC/TMD consortium network* and orofacial pain special interest group†. J Oral Facial Pain Headache 2014;28(1):6–27.

19. Headache classification committee of the international headache society (IHS) the international classification of headache disorders, 3rd edition. Cephalalgia 2018;38(1):1–211.

20. Munksgaard SB, Jensen RH. Medication overuse headache. Headache 2014; 54(7):1251–7.

21. Fernandes G, Siqueira JT, Godoi Gonçalves DA, et al. Association between painful temporomandibular disorders, sleep bruxism and tinnitus. Braz Oral Res 2014;28(1):1–7.

22. Hosoya H, Kitaura H, Hashimoto T, et al. Relationship between sleep bruxism and sleep respiratory events in patients with obstructive sleep apnea syndrome. Sleep Breath 2014;18(4):1–8.

23. Sanders AE, Essick GK, Fillingim R, et al. Sleep apnea symptoms and risk of temporomandibular disorder: OPPERA cohort. J Dent Res 2013;92(7 Suppl): 70S–7S.

24. Neau J-P, Paquereau J, Bailbe M, et al. Relationship between sleep apnoea syndrome, snoring and headaches. Cephalalgia 2002;22(5):333–9.

25. Carlsson GE, Egermark I, Magnusson T. Predictors of signs and symptoms of temporomandibular disorders: a 20-year follow-up study from childhood to adulthood. Acta Odontol Scand 2002;60(3):180–5.

26. Lavigne GJ, Rompré PH, Montplaisir JY, et al. Motor activity in sleep bruxism with concomitant jaw muscle pain. A retrospective pilot study. Eur J Oral Sci 1997; 105(1):92–5.

27. Yachida W, Castrillon EE, Baad-Hansen L, et al. Craniofacial pain and jaw-muscle activity during sleep. J Dent Res 2012;91(6):562–7.

28. Rompré PH, Daigle-Landry D, Guitard F, et al. Identification of a sleep bruxism subgroup with a higher risk of pain. J Dent Res 2007;86(9):837–42.

29. Lund JP, Donga R, Widmer CG, et al. The pain-adaptation model: a discussion of the relationship between chronic musculoskeletal pain and motor activity. Can J Physiol Pharmacol 2011;69(5):683–94.

30. Jadidi F, Castrillon EE, Svensson P. Effect of conditioning electrical stimuli on temporalis electromyographic activity during sleep. J Oral Rehabil 2008;35(3): 171–83.

31. Xu L, Fan S, Cai B, et al. Influence of sustained submaximal clenching fatigue test on electromyographic activity and maximum voluntary bite forces in healthy subjects and patients with temporomandibular disorders. J Oral Rehabil 2017;44(5): 340–6.

32. Takeuchi T, Arima T, Ernberg M, et al. Symptoms and physiological responses to prolonged, repeated, low-level tooth clenching in humans. Headache 2015;55(3): 381–94.

33. Suzuki S, Castrillon EE, Arima T, et al. Blood oxygenation of masseter muscle during sustained elevated muscle activity in healthy participants. J Oral Rehabil 2016;43(12):900–10.

34. Suzuki S, Arima T, Kitagawa Y, et al. Influence of glutamate-evoked pain and sustained elevated muscle activity on blood oxygenation in the human masseter muscle. Eur J Oral Sci 2017;125(6):453–62.

35. Kumar A, Castrillon EE, Svensson KG, et al. Effects of experimental craniofacial pain on fine jaw motor control: a placebo-controlled double-blinded study. Exp Brain Res 2015;233(6):1745–59.

36. Vos T, Flaxman AD, Naghavi M. Erratum: years lived with disability (YLDs) for 1160 sequelae of 289 diseases and injuries 1990-2010: a systematic analysis for the Global Burden of Disease Study 2010. Lancet 2012;380:2163–96. Lancet 2014;384(9943):582.

37. Franco AL, Gonçalves DAG, Castanharo SM, et al. Migraine is the most prevalent primary headache in individuals with temporomandibular disorders. J Oral Facial Pain Headache 2010;24(3):287–92.

38. van der Meer HA, Speksnijder CM, Engelbert RHH, et al. The association between headaches and temporomandibular disorders is confounded by bruxism and somatic symptoms. Clin J Pain 2017;33(9):835–43.

39. Fernandes G, Franco AL, Gonçalves DA, et al. Temporomandibular disorders, sleep bruxism, and primary headaches are mutually associated. J Orofac Pain 2013;27(1):14–20.

40. Franco L, Rompré PH, de Grandmont P, et al. A mandibular advancement appliance reduces pain and rhythmic masticatory muscle activity in patients with morning headache. J Orofac Pain 2011;25(3):240–9.

41. Holmgren K, Sheikholeslam A, Riise C. Effect of a full-arch maxillary occlusal splint on parafunctional activity during sleep in patients with nocturnal bruxism and signs and symptoms of craniomandibular disorders. J Prosthet Dent 1993; 69(3):293–7.

42. Ulfberg J, Carter N, Talbäck M, et al. Headache, snoring and sleep apnoea. J Neurol 1996;243(9):621–5.

43. Göder R, Friege L, Fritzer G, et al. Morning headaches in patients with sleep disorders: a systematic polysomnographic study. Sleep Med 2003;4(5):385–91.

44. Larner AJ. Not all morning headaches are due to brain tumours. Pract Neurol 2009;9(2):80–4.

Sex, Gender, and Orofacial Pain

Jeffry Rowland Shaefer, DDS, MS, MPH[a],*, Shehryar Nasir Khawaja, BDS, MSc[b],
Paula Furlan Bavia, DDS, PhD[c]

KEYWORDS

• Gender • Orofacial pain • Pain perception • Pain modulation • Pain threshold

KEY POINTS

• The female gender has a higher prevalence for almost all pain problems affecting the head, neck, and orofacial pain regions. Trigeminal autonomic cephalalgias and glossopharyngeal neuralgias are exceptions.
• Gender differences in pain thresholds, temporal summation, pain expectations, and somatic awareness exist in patients with chronic temporomandibular disorders (TMD) or orofacial pain.
• Genetic studies indicate that the genetic contribution to the development of TMD and orofacial pain is a small part of the overall risk for these disorders. However, female gender is the most significant risk factor.
• Future research needs to elucidate the sex effects on factors that protect against developing pain or prevent pain from becoming debilitating.
• Specific gender-based treatments for TMD and orofacial pain treatment will evolve from translational research, providing a better understanding of the gender differences in pain modulation and perception.

INTRODUCTION

Orofacial pain is a broad term that comprises multiple painful conditions affecting the oral, head, face, and neck area. Such conditions can involve different structures and be derived from musculoskeletal, vascular, neurovascular, neuropathic, idiopathic, and psychogenic origins.[1] They are very often associated with complex signs and symptoms, which in turn represent a challenge to establish the differential diagnosis

Disclosure Statement: The authors have nothing to disclose.
[a] Division of Oral and Maxillofacial Pain, Department of Oral and Maxillofacial Surgery, Massachusetts General Hospital, Harvard School of Dental Medicine, 55 Fruit Street, Boston, MA 02114, USA; [b] Department of Internal Medicine, Shaukat Khanum Memorial Cancer Hospital, 7A Block R-3 M.A. Johar Town, Lahore, Punjab, Pakistan; [c] Division of Oral and Maxillofacial Pain, Department of Oral and Maxillofacial Surgery, Massachusetts General Hospital, 55 Fruit Street, Boston, MA 02114, USA
* Corresponding author. 4 Monument Circle, Hingham, MA 02043.
E-mail address: jshaefer@mgh.harvard.edu

and the following treatment. Multiple diagnoses are commonly observed in individuals with orofacial pain. Thus, understanding the most common types of pain affecting the orofacial region, as well as their clinical presentation and prevalence in the general population, will assist the clinician to arrive at the most definitive diagnosis.

Evidence shows that painful conditions in the oral and maxillofacial region are relatively common, affecting approximately 10% to 26% of the adult population.[2,3] Several studies demonstrated that such conditions, including but not limited to temporomandibular disorders (TMD), primary headaches, and neuropathic conditions, are highly predominant in women.[2-5] It has also been reported that women seek treatment more often than men with an approximate 2:1 ratio.[4,5] In addition, it is widely believed that pain in general affects men and women differently due to a variety of factors, which must be taken into account during the clinical assessment and treatment.

EPIDEMIOLOGY OF OROFACIAL PAIN
Temporomandibular Disorders

TMD is reported as the most prevalent type of chronic orofacial pain. It comprises a variety of conditions that can affect temporomandibular joints (TMJ), facial, head, and cervical structures. It involves TMJ sounds and restricted jaw movements.[6] Pain in the masticatory musculature is reported by most TMD patients, significantly impairing jaw function.[4] Evidence has shown that TMD is highly prevalent in adulthood, affecting 5% to 12% of the population,[7] and is approximately 3 times more common in women than in men.[8-10] With regards to the TMD subgroups, masticatory myofascial pain disorders are reported in about 45.3% of the TMD patients, followed by disc displacement (41.1%) and other joint disorders (30.1%), with TMJ arthralgia occurring in about 34.2% of the subjects.[10] In addition, there is a high predilection for female gender in all subgroups of TMD, especially those of muscular origin.[11-13] Interestingly, most patients suffering from these disorders often report pain involving other structures, such as in the cervical and head regions. Therefore, because gender does affect the presentation of TMDs, it is imperative to also understand the gender disparity among cervical and headache disorders.

Cervicalgia and Cervicogenic Headache

Cervicalgia is a broad term that refers to pain in the neck region, which is highly prevalent in the world population, with an estimate range from 16.7% to 75.1%.[14] The prevalence of neck pain increases proportionally with age, affecting 27.2% of women and 17.4% of men.[15] Neck pain may be related to any cervical structure; however, most often the discomfort is present in the suboccipital, sternocleidomastoid, and trapezius muscles with a common referred pain to other areas, including frontal, temporoparietal, occipital, vertex, and orbital regions. In addition, cervical pain is very often associated with cervicogenic headaches,[16] which are estimated to affect 0.4% to 2.5% of the general population and about 15% to 20% of subjects with chronic headaches. Equally, women, with a female-to-male ratio of 4:1, more often report this condition.[17]

Headache Attributed to Giant Cell Arteritis

Giant cell arteritis (GCA) is the most common primary systemic vasculitis,[18] characterized by several important manifestations, including headache, fever, polymyalgia rheumatica, and visual disturbances.[19] In addition, patients with this condition typically experience pain in the head, face, and neck region, with jaw claudication a particular orofacial symptom associated with GCA. This condition primarily affects the elderly population, and the incidence begins at the fifth decade, increasing with age, with a peak incidence around the age of 70 or 80 years.[19] GCA incidence is higher in Scandinavian countries, varying from 10 to 20/100,000 cases per year.[20–23] Recent evidence has shown that women are about 3 times more affected with this condition than men.[24]

Primary Headache Disorders

Tension-type headache and migraine
Tension-type headache (TTH) is the most common form of all primary headaches. With lifetime prevalence greater than 80%,[25] this condition is experienced by most individuals at least once in life. TTH occurs mainly between 20 and 40 years of age, with a high prevalence in the fifth decade of life.[26] In addition, the 1-year prevalence rate for TTH has been reported in 86% of women and 63% of men.[27] Similarly, a more recent study demonstrated that episodic TTH affects 71.6% of women and 49% of men, with a female-to-male ratio of 1.5:1.[28] Moreover, it has been reported that the episodic form is relatively influenced by environmental factors,[29] whereas chronic TTH is highly predisposed by a genetic component.[30] Likewise, environment and genetics are largely associated with migraine disorders, in which first-degree relatives are twice and 4 times more likely to experience migraine without and with aura, respectively.[31] At least 12% of the general population and approximately 36 million Americans suffer from migraines.[32] There is a high predilection for female gender, especially with regards to episodic migraine, which occurs in about 18% of women and 6% of men,[32,33] with a female-to-male ratio on the order of 3:1. It has been reported that the female preponderance in migraine headaches is also possibly linked to hormonal factors. In addition, women very often present higher rates of most migraine symptoms, including aura, greater associated impairment, and higher health care utilization than men.[33]

Trigeminal autonomic cephalalgias
Different than TTH and migraine, trigeminal autonomic cephalalgias (TAC) are fairly uncommon forms of headaches, with a male predilection. It is well known that cluster headache is the most severe of the primary headaches. Moreover, it is the most common type of TAC, with a 1-year prevalence of approximately 0.53%[34,35] and a marked preponderance in men, with a male-to-female ratio varying from 3.3:1 to approximately 8.4:1.[36] The gender disparity seems to be associated with lifestyle, and tobacco and alcohol use have been cited as possible triggering factors in cluster headache sufferers.[34,37] Furthermore, there is also a hereditary propensity, with first-degree relatives being up to 39 times more subjected to develop cluster headaches.[38,39] Short-lasting unilateral neuralgiform headache with conjunctival injection and tearing (SUNCT) is another rare condition, with an incidence and prevalence of about 1.2 and 6.6/100,000, respectively.[40] The male predilection was primarily reported with an estimated male-to-female ratio of 7:1[41]; however, with an ascending number of female cases, this condition is currently considered to be only slightly more common in men, about 1.5:1.[42] Paroxysmal hemicrania is an extremely rare disorder, and its prevalence has been estimated in 0.02% to 0.07%, predominantly in women with a female-to-male ratio of nearly 1.6:1.[43] Likewise, hemicrania continua is a form of infrequent headache occurring in about 1% of the population, with most cases reported in women (female-to-male ratio, 2.8:1).[44,45]

Neuropathic Pain Conditions

Trigeminal neuralgia

Trigeminal neuralgia (TN) is a neuropathic pain disorder considered one of the most painful conditions involving the orofacial region.[46] Classical TN represents 80% to 90% of TN cases and has unremarkable clinical and imaging findings.[47] The term symptomatic (or secondary) accounts for the minority of patients, and the symptoms are secondary to another neurologic disease or trauma involving the trigeminal system. TN is considered a rare condition, and its prevalence is poorly reported. Evidence estimates an incidence of 4.3 to 27 cases of TN per 100,000 per year,[48,49] more common in individuals older than 60 years. In addition, TN more frequently affects women,[50] with an annual occurrence of approximately 5.9/100,000 cases per women and nearly 3.4/100,000 cases per men,[48] with a female-to-male proportion of 1.6:1.[51]

Glossopharyngeal neuralgia

Glossopharyngeal neuralgia is an extremely rare neuralgiform disorder responsible for pain involving pharynx, tonsil, soft palate, and posterior tongue base with possible radiation to the inner ear or angle of the mandible.[46] It occurs much less frequently than TN with an incidence estimated at 0.2 to 0.4/100,000 persons per year.[52] Similar to TN, this condition also affects individuals older than 50 years and increases with age. On the other hand, there is no gender predilection, and glossopharyngeal neuralgia appears to be equally distributed in women and men.[53]

Burning mouth syndrome

Burning mouth syndrome (BMS), another form of neuropathy, is characterized by burning pain localized in the tongue and oral mucosa often without evident clinical signs. It may be associated with subjective dryness of the mouth, sensations of dysesthesia, and taste disturbances.[46] BMS is not an uncommon condition and affects about 0.7% to 15% of the general population, especially affecting middle-aged postmenopausal women.[54] It occurs usually in the fifth and seventh decades, and the prevalence increases directly proportionally with age in both genders; however, BMS tends to occur approximately 7 times more in women than men.[55]

SEX, GENDER, AND PAIN

It is well established that sex differences in pain exist. The underlying pathophysiology is complex and unclear. However, it has been proposed that gender effects on pain are from an interaction of biological, psychological, and sociocultural factors.

SEX AND PAIN

Hormones and Pain

Gonadal hormones play an important role in the reproductive system. In women, estrogens and progesterone levels alter through the course of menstrual cycle, during pregnancy, and after menopause. Alternatively, in men, testosterone levels deteriorate with aging. Data on the association of gonadal hormones with pain are inconsistent, and what association exists is convoluted by the presence of methodological disparities and deficiencies in the studies that support the association. Studies in animals have relied on different nociceptive assays (electrical, thermal, chemical) and measurement responses (tail flick, jump, behavioral cries). Furthermore, the temporal characteristics used in these studies, such as duration and intensity of nociceptive stimulation, vary.[56–58] Nonetheless, current literature based on animal-model studies and human-based investigations suggests that conditions characterized by elevated estrogens either alone, or in association with increased progesterone levels, are associated with increased sensitivity to nociception, or diminished analgesic response to stress and opioid medications. However, there are exceptions, because elevated estrogens and progesterone levels can also inhibit nociceptive pathways and potentiate k-opioid analgesia, such as during the third trimester of pregnancy.[56,57]

Hormonal modulation of pain is complex. Hormones influence the peripheral and central nervous system events at various steps of nociceptive process and are considered to have a significant contribution to the sex differences in pain.[57]

Raised estrogen levels can result in enlargement of the receptive field of peripheral nociceptors in the trigeminal system. These changes are similar to those observed after both chemical and surgical sympathectomy. However, this does not alter the threshold required to activate peripheral nociceptors.[59] Likewise, multiple investigations have suggested that in periods of high levels of progesterone, such as during pregnancy, nerve conduction is altered, and the susceptibility of both somatic and visceral peripheral nerves to the effects of local anesthetics increases.[60,61]

Gonadal hormones can influence the process of peripheral sensitization. Alteration in the level of hormones was associated with activation of "silent" nociceptors such as those that exist in the TMJ capsule.[62,63] It has been suggested that variation in hormonal levels influence nerve growth factor (NGF) and its high affinity receptors, *trk A*. Studies have found upregulation of *trk A* messenger RNA (mRNA) expression in dorsal root ganglions during the course of menstrual cycle. Once activated, NGF can initiate and promote neurite sprouting and fiber growth.[62,63] Likewise, estrogens may modulate the activity of the bradykinin B2 receptor and alter the concentration of various neuromodulators that are directly or indirectly involved in its nociceptive pathway, such as substance P, glutamate, gamma-aminobutyric acid, dopamine, serotonin, and epinephrine.[56,57]

Estrogens and progesterone levels also affect the endogenous opioid system and the cholinergic system. It has been reported that women in high estradiol states exhibit reduced pain sensitivity and increased brain mu-opioid binding. Opposite results were reported for women in low estradiol states.[64] Estrogens and progesterone influence the concentration of luteinizing hormone (LH) through a negative feedback mechanism. At high levels, they cause the pituitary gland to decrease secretion of LH. LH results in downregulation of central opioid receptors and has been associated with a reduction in opioid response.[65] Similarly, gonadal hormones affect the central cholinergic system. Investigations have found estrogen-dependent increases in the brain, in the activity of choline acetyltransferase mRNA enzymatic activity and high-affinity choline uptake, to result in increased acetylcholine release.[66]

Furthermore, there are multiple excitatory and inhibitory mechanisms through which hormones may directly or indirectly modulate the nociceptive response. These modulations include decreased sensorimotor inhibition, sleep disturbances, and behavioral and affective states.[57]

Animal-based investigations using carrageenan-induced mechanical allodynia, lumbar nerve injury-induced mechanical allodynia, and the thermal hyperalgesia model for pain have suggested that neonatal exposure to testosterone results in lesser sensitivity to noxious stimuli. Likewise, NMDA-mediated stress-induced antinociception has been shown to depend on neonatal exposure to testosterone.[56] Contrary to these findings, there are reports of failure of testosterone manipulations to reverse or eradicate sex differences in nociception.[56,67] This conflict may be explained by the methodological differences present in these investigations.

Analogous changes have been observed in clinical studies. Nearly half of the patients undergoing female-to-male hormonal treatment with testosterone were found to have a significant improvement in symptoms associated with chronic headache disorder. Similarly, testosterone level has been reported to be a key variable in modulating pain sensitivity in women that are in a low endogenous estradiol state (using oral contraceptives).[56] Furthermore, brain imaging has suggested that patients with low levels of testosterone are unable to engage descending inhibition at the level of the rostral ventromedial medulla.[56,68]

Genetics and Pain

There is cumulative evidence present in the literature that suggests genetics to be a contributing factor for sex-related differences in pain. Genetics can influence the nociceptive sensitivity, pathways, and perception. A study based on healthy human volunteers found A118G single nucleotide polymorphism, a common variant of the mu-opioid receptor gene (OPRM 1), was associated with greater pressure pain thresholds than those with homozygous alleles. In addition, presence of a polymorphism was found to be associated with thermal pain perception. However, this association was in a sex-dependent manner. In women, it was associated with pain sensitivity, whereas the opposite affect was observed for men.[69] Similar results have been reported in clinical investigations. Women with this rare allele experienced poorer recovery from lumbar disc herniation and radicular pain, whereas presence of A118G single nucleotide polymorphism was associated with enhanced recovery among men.[70,71] On the contrary, presence of A118G was associated with early recovery and less pain in women following motor vehicle accident when compared with men.[72]

Presence of melanocortin-1 receptor (Mc1r) gene, associated with the presence of red hair and fair skin, was reported to be associated with analgesia in a sex-dependent manner. Women with 2 variant alleles of MC1R displayed greater analgesic response from kappa-opioid (pentazocine) relative to men and women with other allele variants.[73]

Catechol-O-methyltransferase (COMT) enzyme regulates activity of catechol-containing compounds, such as epinephrine, norepinephrine, and dopamine. It is an important regulator of neurotransmitters involved in various neurologic functions, including pain perception and mood.[74] Multiple single nucleotide polymorphisms associated with COMT have been identified. Findings from these investigations have identified 3 COMT haplotypes, a low pain sensitivity (LPS), average pain sensitivity, and high pain sensitivity (HPS) haplotype. HPS and LPS have been found to be associated with generalized increased and reduced risk of developing a chronic pain condition, respectively. However, recently a sex-dependent difference of COMT genetic variant on pain sensitivity was identified. Investigators reported an association between HPS haplotype, sex, and stress in a post–motor vehicle collision cohort. Furthermore, it was found that women reported higher pain sensitivity than men, at the same epinephrine level.[75]

Similar findings have been reported for single nucleotide polymorphism of Avpr1a gene, encoding for vasopressin-1 A (V1AR) receptor. Vasopressin is involved in activation of endogenous analgesia. Multiple animal-model investigations, as well as clinical human-based studies, have suggested a male-specific interaction between stress, pain, and a single nucleotide polymorphism of the Avpr1a gene.[76]

Resting Blood Pressure and Pain

Resting blood pressure has been associated inversely with pain sensitivity and proportionally with pain threshold in individuals with no history of chronic pain disorder and hypertension.[77] Some of the investigators have reported sex-dependent differences in this effect and suggested that it may partially account for the sex-related differences in pain.[78,79] Women are reported to have a higher pain threshold compared with men for experimental pain stimuli. However, the magnitude of the differences was not significant to independently account for sex-related differences in pain.[79] Similarly, other investigators have not reported any sex-dependent difference in association between pain sensitivity, pain threshold, and resting blood pressure.[77,80]

GENDER AND PAIN

As mentioned earlier, sex refers to biological distinctions characterizing men and women. On the contrary, gender alludes to sex-related social roles with which an individual identifies.[67] Gender may influence sex-related differences in pain, through sociocultural and psychological characteristics.

Masculinity, Femininity, and Pain

Multiple investigations have been conducted on the association of masculinity, femininity, and pain response.[67,79] Experimental pain studies have suggested that sex-related differences exist in association with the level of masculinity and mechanical pain threshold.[67,81,82] Men with a higher concept of self-masculinity reported greater mechanical pain thresholds. Similarly, in both women and men, masculinity was found to be associated with higher mechanical pain tolerance.[67,81] However, contrary to mechanical pain–based experimental studies, investigations using cold pain have reported conflicting findings. Where some investigators have reported femininity to be associated with lower cold pain tolerance, others have found an association of higher masculinity in comparison to femininity to be associated with higher cold pain tolerance and lower cold pain ratings.[67,79,81,82]

Gender Role and Pain

Gender role determined in a society and culture may affect the sex-related differences in pain. It has been reported that women view overt pain expression as more acceptable than men, and these beliefs were predictive of cold pain tolerance.[67,81] Likewise, another group of investigators found both men and women believed that the ideal man should be more tolerant to pain than the ideal woman, and the degree of acceptance to this ideation was associated with greater electrical pain tolerance among men.[83] Correspondingly, it has been reported that women are more willing to report pain than men, and that this perception was found to be associated with sex-related difference in heat pain threshold and tolerance. However, after controlling for willingness to report pain, the difference in heat pain threshold was no longer statistically significant. Nevertheless, sex-related difference in heat pain tolerance persisted.[84]

    Investigations measuring the role of gender-related expectations found that men reported less cold pressor pain, higher pressure pain thresholds,[85] lower heat pain, lower ratings of arousal, and higher cold tolerance,[86] in the presence of a female versus a male experimenter. On the contrary, no such differences were observed in women, except for cold pain tolerance. Women reported higher tolerance to cold pain stimulation in the presence of men.[67,86] Similarly, men reported higher tolerance to ischemic pain after being informed that the female gender was able to tolerate the procedure better.[67] Interestingly, women reported higher tolerance when informed that the female gender had tolerated this procedure better.[87]

Psychological Factors and Pain

Cognitive and affective factors have been suggested to influence pain responses. However, the magnitude of this association is uncertain. Several investigations have suggested that sex-related differences exist in pain coping. Women have been reported to rely on more coping strategies than men, including positive self-statements, problem-focused coping, and use of more social and emotional support. However, they also exhibit higher levels of catastrophizing, and more complex behavioral patterns.[67,81,88]

Affective distress (in form of anxiety), a negative behavioral and emotional consequence to a perceived or real threat, anxiety sensitivity, a fear of anxiety-related bodily sensations,[89] and depression, a condition in which a person feels discouraged, sad, hopeless, unmotivated, or disinterested in life,[90] have been associated with pain in experimental and clinical-based investigations.[67,81,90] Experimental-based pain investigations found anxiety to be positively associated with pain sensitivity among men. However, no such associations were reported for women.[67,81,91] Similar results have been reported in clinical-based studies.[67,81,92] On the contrary, anxiety

Table 1
Sex prevalence in pain disorders

Female Prevalence	Male Prevalence	No Sex Prevalence
Head and Neck Pain		
Migraine headache with aura	Migraine without aura	Acute tension headache
Chronic tension headache	Cluster headache	Cluster-tic syndrome
Postdural puncture headache	Posttraumatic headache	"Jabs" and "jolts" syndrome
Hemicrania continua	SUNCT syndrome	Secondary TN
Cervicogenic headache	Raeder paratrigeminal	Nervus intermedius neuralgia
Tic douloureux	syndrome	Painful ophthalmoplegia
TMJ disorder		Toothache due to pulpitis
Occipital neuralgia		Cracked tooth syndrome
Periapical periodontitis & abscess		Dry socket
Atypical odontalgia		Vagus nerve neuralgia
Burning tongue		Stylohyoid process syndrome
Carotidynia		
Chronic paroxysmal hemicrania		
Temporal arteritis		
Generalized Syndromes		
Carpal tunnel syndrome	Ankylosing spondylitis	Thoracic outlet syndrome
Raynaud disease	Pancreatic disease	Familial Mediterranean fever
Chilblains	Lateral femoral cutaneous	Acute herpes zoster
Causalgia	neuropathy	
Reflex sympathetic dystrophy	Postherpetic neuralgia	
Multiple sclerosis	Hemophilic arthropathy	
Rheumatoid arthritis	Brachial plexus avulsion	
Pain of psychological origin	Lateral femoral cutaneous	
	neuropathy	
Visceral Pain		
Irritable bowel syndrome	Abdominal migraine	Esophageal motility disorders
Interstitial cystitis	Duodenal ulcer	Chronic gastric ulcer
Twelfth rib syndrome		Crohn's disease
Gallbladder disease		Diverticular disease of colon
Chronic constipation		Carcinoma of the colon
Pyriformis syndrome		

From Berkley KJ. Sex differences in pain. Behav Brain Sci 1997;20:371–80; with permission.

Table 2
Gender-related drug pharmacokinetic and pharmacodynamic effects

Drug	Action	Result	Pathway	Reference
Antiepileptics				
Carbamazipine	Decreased level of contraceptive steroids (oral contraceptive [OCI])	Breakthrough bleeding Ovulation	Rapid inducer of P450 system known to decrease levels OC	Davis et al,[107] 2011
Lamotrigine (LTG) and oxcarbazepine (OXC)	During pregnancy clearance of LTG/ OXC is altered	Increase in seizures	Increased excretion explained by steroid induction of hepatic N-2 glucuronidation	Wegner et al,[117] 2010
Muscle Relaxants				
Tizanidine	"Any possible effect of gender and smoking is largely outweighed by individual variability in CYP1A2 activity due to genetic and environmental factors and in body weight. Careful dosing of tizanidine is warranted in small females, whereas male smokers can require higher than average doses"	Mean values of C_{max} (the peak plasma concentration) and $AUC_{0-\infty}$ (the area under plasma concentrations from 0 to infinity) were 30% and 34% higher in women than in men, and in 5 of the 18 women, the C_{max} of tizanidine was higher than in any men. However, the mean elimination $t_{1/2}$ of tizanidine was 9% shorter in the non-smoking women than non-smoking men	Men > cytochrome P450 (CYP) isoenzymes, for example, CYP1A2 and CYP2E1, but < CYP3A4. Differences in the membrane transport of exogenous compounds exist ≥ excretion of pravastatin in men (single nucleotide polymorphism in hepatic uptake transporter organic anion transporting polypeptide 1B1). Women < glomerular filtration rate	Backman et al,[104] 2008

(continued on next page)

Table 2
(continued)

Drug	Action	Result	Pathway	Reference
Tizanidine	Effect of combined OCs on CYP1A2 activity (inhibition)	OCs containing ethinylestradiol and gestodene increase the plasma concentrations of tizanidine	CYP1A2. Care should be exercised when tizanidine is prescribed to OC users	Granfors et al,[110] 2005
Tocolytic agents (prevention of premature birth)	Pharmacologic agents used to treat preterm labor (review); includes beta-adrenergic agonists, nonsteroidal anti-inflammatory drugs (NSAIDs), calcium channel blockers, magnesium sulfate, oxytocin agonists	During pregnancy: Oral absorption < due to delayed stomach emptying and < intestinal motility. The volume of distribution of drugs >. Liver metabolic activity >, Renal filtration >. Result: reduced plasma concentration and reduced half-life of most drugs in pregnant women	NSAIDs (indomethacin specifically) was the first choice to prevent preterm delivery, but 100% placental transfer, 7-fold > in fetal half-life, and premature closure of the ductus arteriosus no longer used as a tocolytic agent	Tsatsaris et al,[115] 2004
NSAIDs				
Keterolac (low dose)	Gender was not really a factor in this study; all subjects were women			Bendixen et al,[105,106] 2010
Ibuprofen	Can cause hypersensitivity reaction. The highest incidence of liver reaction is seen in women. Women >50 are at higher risk than men	Hypersensitivity reaction and liver damage	Ibuprofen inhibits cyclooxygenase-1 (COX-1) & COX-2 by 50% Variability in CP450, CYP2C9, and CYP2C8 can affect metabolism of NSAIDs	Nanau and Neuman,[114] 2010
Opioids				
Methadone	Rate of clearance of methadone during pregnancy changes	As pregnancy progresses, addicted patients may need smaller or larger doses	The induction effect of liver enzymes CYP3A4 and CYP2D6, typically noninducible, effect metabolism	Wolff et al,[118] 2005

Drug	Pharmacokinetics	Nonpharmacokinetic factors	Clinical notes	Reference
Tramadol	Pharmacokinetics of tramadol and its metabolites		No significant gender differences pharmacokinetics of tramadol	Ardakani & Rouini,[103] 2007
Sedatives and Hypnotics				
Triazolam	CYP4503A		Gender differences in triazolam kinetics were not apparent; there were age differences	Greenblatt et al,[111] 2004
Triptans	Numerous kinetic parameters of triptans vary according to gender. C_{max} and $AUC_{0-\infty}$ of frovatriptan, naratriptan, rizatriptan, and zolmitriptan are < in men due to higher bioavailability in women and > total body clearance in men	Nonpharmacokinetic factors of variability of response to triptans: • Genetic polymorphisms • Receptor adaptation • Fluctuation of migraine • Prophylactic treatments • Previous therapies • Time of medication • Severity of migraine attack	Wide variance in response to explain triptan efficacy	Ferrari et al,[109] 2011
Sumatriptan	Studied times to response and therapeutic threshold with either response or no response to sumatriptan	Wide variability in plasma concentrations after oral dose in both sexes. Also high variability with fast-disintegrating formulation	Intersubject variability in plasma concentration after subcutaneous use clinically nonsignificant	Ferrari et al,[108] 2008
Frovitriptan	Women OC users had 26%–68% higher C_{max} and AUC		Twice daily lower dose recommended to maintain therapeutic levels to prevent menstrual migraine	Wade et al,[116] 2009
Selective serotonin reuptake inhibitors				
Duloxetine	CYP2D6 enzyme is involved in the metabolism of duloxetine. CYP1A2 activity is higher in men and smokers than in women and non-smokers	Other CYP enzymes implicated. Tested CYP1A2 enzymes involved in duloxetine metabolism	Duloxetine did not clinically affect CYP1A2 levels, but coadministration of duloxetine with potent CYP1A2 inhibitors should be avoided	Lobo et al,[112] 2008
Duloxetine	Reduced stress, urinary incontinence in women	All subjects were women		McCormack & Keating,[113] 2004

sensitivity was concluded to be higher among women and associated with pain-related sex differences in various clinical and experimental-based investigations.[93–96] Also, gender was reported to influence the association between chronic pain disorders and depression. Gender was reported to positively influence the relationship between depression and pain, in men, but not in women.[81,97] Similarly, in individuals with depression, women are more likely than men to report chronic pain.[67,81,98]

SUMMARY

The female gender has a higher prevalence for almost all pain problems (**Table 1**) affecting the head, neck, and orofacial pain regions. TACs and glossopharyngeal neuralgias are exceptions. Genetic studies indicate that the genetic contribution to the development of TMD and orofacial pain is a small part of the overall risk for these disorders. However, female gender is the single biggest risk factor.[99] It must be realized that gender differences in pain thresholds, temporal summation, pain expectations, and somatic awareness exist in patients with chronic TMD or orofacial pain.[100,101] Because of these gender differences, it is recommended that investigators performing medication trials report outcomes for each sex[102] (**Table 2**). Future research also needs to elucidate gender effects on factors that protect against developing pain or preventing pain from becoming debilitating.[100] However, one needs to remember that there are indications that individuals, no matter their gender, who present with chronic orofacial pain have similar genetic, psychological, and behavioral influences affecting pain processing and perception, that is, if they have chronic orofacial pain, there exists a likelihood it is related to a pain-processing deficiency, leading to sensitization or an inability to modulate pain.[99] Further understanding is needed of the impact of pain and trauma on infants, children, and adolescents and how a history of such early trauma contributes to pain sensitivity and response to reinjure in adulthood.[100,101] Such knowledge can then be used to improve pain management for both sexes and should result in specific gender-based treatments for TMD and orofacial pain treatment.

REFERENCES

1. Sarlani E, Balciunas BA, Grace EG. Orofacial pain–part i: assessment and management of musculoskeletal and neuropathic causes. AACN Clin Issues 2005; 16(3):333–46.
2. Madland G, Newton-John T, Feinmann C. Chronic idiopathic orofacial pain: I: what is the evidence base? Br Dent J 2001;191(1):22–4.
3. Macfarlane TV, Blinkhorn AS, Davies RM, et al. Association between local mechanical factors and orofacial pain: survey in the community. J Dent 2003; 31(8):535–42.
4. Dao TT, LeResche L. Gender differences in pain. J Orofac Pain 2000;14(3): 169–84 [discussion: 184–95].
5. Fillingim RB. Sex, gender, and pain: women and men really are different. Curr Rev Pain 2000;4(1):24–30.
6. Cooper BC, Kleinberg I. Examination of a large patient population for the presence of symptoms and signs of temporomandibular disorders. Cranio 2007; 25(2):114–26.
7. Pain.NIoDaCRF. Available at: http://www.nidcr.nih.gov/DataStatistics/FindData ByTopic/FacialPain. Accessed November 15, 2017.
8. LeResche L. Epidemiology of temporomandibular disorders: implications for the investigation of etiologic factors. Crit Rev Oral Biol Med 1997;8(3):291–305.

9. Anastassaki Kohler A, Hugoson A, Magnusson T. Prevalence of symptoms indicative of temporomandibular disorders in adults: cross-sectional epidemiological investigations covering two decades. Acta Odontol Scand 2012;70(3): 213–23.

10. Manfredini D, Guarda-Nardini L, Winocur E, et al. Research diagnostic criteria for temporomandibular disorders: a systematic review of axis I epidemiologic findings. Oral Surg Oral Med Oral Pathol Oral Radiol Endod 2011;112(4): 453–62.

11. Blanco-Hungria A, Blanco-Aguilera A, Blanco-Aguilera E, et al. Prevalence of the different Axis I clinical subtypes in a sample of patients with orofacial pain and temporomandibular disorders in the Andalusian Healthcare Service. Med Oral Patol Oral Cir Bucal 2016;21(2):e169–77.

12. Johansson A, Unell L, Carlsson GE, et al. Gender difference in symptoms related to temporomandibular disorders in a population of 50-year-old subjects. J Orofac Pain 2003;17(1):29–35.

13. Bagis B, Ayaz EA, Turgut S, et al. Gender difference in prevalence of signs and symptoms of temporomandibular joint disorders: a retrospective study on 243 consecutive patients. Int J Med Sci 2012;9(7):539–44.

14. Fejer R, Kyvik KO, Hartvigsen J. The prevalence of neck pain in the world population: a systematic critical review of the literature. Eur Spine J 2006;15(6): 834–48.

15. Hoy DG, Protani M, De R, et al. The epidemiology of neck pain. Best Pract Res Clin Rheumatol 2010;24(6):783–92.

16. Sjaastad O, Wang H, Bakketeig LS. Neck pain and associated head pain: persistent neck complaint with subsequent, transient, posterior headache. Acta Neurol Scand 2006;114(6):392–9.

17. Haldeman S, Dagenais S. Cervicogenic headaches: a critical review. Spine J 2001;1(1):31–46.

18. Romero-Gomez C, Aguilar-Garcia JA, Garcia-de-Lucas MD, et al. Epidemiological study of primary systemic vasculitides among adults in southern Spain and review of the main epidemiological studies. Clin Exp Rheumatol 2015;33(2 Suppl 89):S-11-18.

19. Nesher G. The diagnosis and classification of giant cell arteritis. J Autoimmun 2014;48–49:73–5.

20. Salvarani C, Macchioni P, Zizzi F, et al. Epidemiologic and immunogenetic aspects of polymyalgia rheumatica and giant cell arteritis in northern Italy. Arthritis Rheum 1991;34(3):351–6.

21. Salvarani C, Crowson CS, O'Fallon WM, et al. Reappraisal of the epidemiology of giant cell arteritis in Olmsted County, Minnesota, over a fifty-year period. Arthritis Rheum 2004;51(2):264–8.

22. Gonzalez-Gay MA, Miranda-Filloy JA, Lopez-Diaz MJ, et al. Giant cell arteritis in northwestern Spain: a 25-year epidemiologic study. Medicine (Baltimore) 2007; 86(2):61–8.

23. Haugeberg G, Paulsen PQ, Bie RB. Temporal arteritis in Vest Agder County in southern Norway: incidence and clinical findings. J Rheumatol 2000;27(11): 2624–7.

24. Sturm A, Dechant C, Proft F, et al. Gender differences in giant cell arteritis: a case-control study. Clin Exp Rheumatol 2016;34(3 Suppl 97):S70–2.

25. Lyngberg AC, Rasmussen BK, Jorgensen T, et al. Incidence of primary headache: a Danish epidemiologic follow-up study. Am J Epidemiol 2005;161(11): 1066–73.

26. Lyngberg AC, Rasmussen BK, Jorgensen T, et al. Has the prevalence of migraine and tension-type headache changed over a 12-year period? A Danish population survey. Eur J Epidemiol 2005;20(3):243–9.

27. Rasmussen BK, Jensen R, Schroll M, et al. Epidemiology of headache in a general population–a prevalence study. J Clin Epidemiol 1991;44(11):1147–57.

28. Lebedeva ER, Kobzeva NR, Gilev D, et al. Prevalence of primary headache disorders diagnosed according to ICHD-3 beta in three different social groups. Cephalalgia 2016;36(6):579–88.

29. Ulrich V, Gervil M, Olesen J. The relative influence of environment and genes in episodic tension-type headache. Neurology 2004;62(11):2065–9.

30. Ostergaard S, Russell MB, Bendtsen L, et al. Comparison of first degree relatives and spouses of people with chronic tension headache. BMJ 1997; 314(7087):1092–3.

31. Russell MB, Iselius L, Olesen J. Migraine without aura and migraine with aura are inherited disorders. Cephalalgia 1996;16(5):305–9.

32. Lipton RB, Bigal ME, Diamond M, et al. Migraine prevalence, disease burden, and the need for preventive therapy. Neurology 2007;68(5):343–9.

33. Buse DC, Loder EW, Gorman JA, et al. Sex differences in the prevalence, symptoms, and associated features of migraine, probable migraine and other severe headache: results of the American Migraine Prevalence and Prevention (AMPP) study. Headache 2013;53(8):1278–99.

34. Robbins MS, Lipton RB. The epidemiology of primary headache disorders. Semin Neurol 2010;30(2):107–19.

35. Fischera M, Marziniak M, Gralow I, et al. The incidence and prevalence of cluster headache: a meta-analysis of population-based studies. Cephalalgia 2008; 28(6):614–8.

36. Ekbom K, Svensson DA, Traff H, et al. Age at onset and sex ratio in cluster headache: observations over three decades. Cephalalgia 2002;22(2):94–100.

37. May A. Cluster headache: pathogenesis, diagnosis, and management. Lancet 2005;366(9488):843–55.

38. Leone M, Russell MB, Rigamonti A, et al. Increased familial risk of cluster headache. Neurology 2001;56(9):1233–6.

39. Russell MB. Epidemiology and genetics of cluster headache. Lancet Neurol 2004;3(5):279–83.

40. Williams MH, Broadley SA. SUNCT and SUNA: clinical features and medical treatment. J Clin Neurosci 2008;15(5):526–34.

41. Benoliel R, Sharav Y. SUNCT syndrome: case report and literature review. Oral Surg Oral Med Oral Pathol Oral Radiol Endod 1998;85(2):158–61.

42. Matharu MS, Cohen AS, Boes CJ, et al. Short-lasting unilateral neuralgiform headache with conjunctival injection and tearing syndrome: a review. Curr Pain Headache Rep 2003;7(4):308–18.

43. Sjaastad O, Bakketeig LS. The rare, unilateral headaches. Vaga study of headache epidemiology. J Headache Pain 2007;8(1):19–27.

44. Peres MF, Silberstein SD, Nahmias S, et al. Hemicrania continua is not that rare. Neurology 2001;57(6):948–51.

45. Obermann M, Katsarava Z. Epidemiology of unilateral headaches. Expert Rev Neurother 2008;8(9):1313–20.

46. Headache Classification Committee of the International Headache Society. The international classification of headache disorders, 3rd edition (beta version). Cephalalgia 2013;33(9):629–808.

47. Love S, Coakham HB. Trigeminal neuralgia: pathology and pathogenesis. Brain 2001;124(Pt 12):2347–60.
48. Katusic S, Beard CM, Bergstralh E, et al. Incidence and clinical features of trigeminal neuralgia, Rochester, Minnesota, 1945-1984. Ann Neurol 1990;27(1): 89–95.
49. Hall GC, Carroll D, McQuay HJ. Primary care incidence and treatment of four neuropathic pain conditions: a descriptive study, 2002-2005. BMC Fam Pract 2008;9:26.
50. Siqueira SR, Teixeira MJ, Siqueira JT. Clinical characteristics of patients with trigeminal neuralgia referred to neurosurgery. Eur J Dent 2009;3(3):207–12.
51. Bennetto L, Patel NK, Fuller G. Trigeminal neuralgia and its management. BMJ 2007;334(7586):201–5.
52. van Hecke O, Austin SK, Khan RA, et al. Neuropathic pain in the general population: a systematic review of epidemiological studies. Pain 2014;155(4): 654–62.
53. Koopman JS, Dieleman JP, Huygen FJ, et al. Incidence of facial pain in the general population. Pain 2009;147(1–3):122–7.
54. Zakrzewska JM, Forssell H, Glenny AM. Interventions for the treatment of burning mouth syndrome. Cochrane Database Syst Rev 2005;(1):CD002779.
55. Nasri-Heir C, Zagury JG, Thomas D, et al. Burning mouth syndrome: current concepts. J Indian Prosthodont Soc 2015;15(4):300–7.
56. Craft RM. Modulation of pain by estrogens. Pain 2007;132(Suppl 1):S3–12.
57. Fillingim RB, Ness TJ. Sex-related hormonal influences on pain and analgesic responses. Neurosci Biobehav Rev 2000;24(4):485–501.
58. Bartley EJ, Fillingim RB. Sex differences in pain: a brief review of clinical and experimental findings. Br J Anaesth 2013;111(1):52–8.
59. Bereiter DA, Stanford LR, Barker DJ. Hormone-induced enlargement of receptive fields in trigeminal mechanoreceptive neurons. II. Possible mechanisms. Brain Res 1980;184(2):411–23.
60. Butterworth JFT, Walker FO, Lysak SZ. Pregnancy increases median nerve susceptibility to lidocaine. Anesthesiology 1990;72(6):962–5.
61. Datta S, Migliozzi RP, Flanagan HL, et al. Chronically administered progesterone decreases halothane requirements in rabbits. Anesth Analg 1989;68(1): 46–50.
62. McMahon SB. NGF as a mediator of inflammatory pain. Philos Trans R Soc Lond B Biol Sci 1996;351(1338):431–40.
63. Sohrabji F, Miranda RC, Toran-Allerand CD. Estrogen differentially regulates estrogen and nerve growth factor receptor mRNAs in adult sensory neurons. J Neurosci 1994;14(2):459–71.
64. Smith YR, Stohler CS, Nichols TE, et al. Pronociceptive and antinociceptive effects of estradiol through endogenous opioid neurotransmission in women. J Neurosci 2006;26(21):5777–85.
65. Lavand'homme PM, Eisenach JC. Sex differences in cholinergic analgesia II: differing mechanisms in two models of allodynia. Anesthesiology 1999;91(5): 1455–61.
66. Chiari A, Tobin JR, Pan HL, et al. Sex differences in cholinergic analgesia I: a supplemental nicotinic mechanism in normal females. Anesthesiology 1999; 91(5):1447–54.
67. Fillingim RB, King CD, Ribeiro-Dasilva MC, et al. Sex, gender, and pain: a review of recent clinical and experimental findings. J Pain 2009;10(5):447–85.

68. Vincent K, Warnaby C, Stagg CJ, et al. Brain imaging reveals that engagement of descending inhibitory pain pathways in healthy women in a low endogenous estradiol state varies with testosterone. Pain 2013;154(4):515–24.

69. Fillingim RB, Kaplan L, Staud R, et al. The A118G single nucleotide polymorphism of the mu-opioid receptor gene (OPRM1) is associated with pressure pain sensitivity in humans. J Pain 2005;6(3):159–67.

70. Olsen MB, Jacobsen LM, Schistad EI, et al. Pain intensity the first year after lumbar disc herniation is associated with the A118G polymorphism in the opioid receptor mu 1 gene: evidence of a sex and genotype interaction. J Neurosci 2012; 32(29):9831–4.

71. Hasvik E, Iordanova Schistad E, Grøvle L, et al. Subjective health complaints in patients with lumbar radicular pain and disc herniation are associated with a sex - OPRM1 A118G polymorphism interaction: a prospective 1-year observational study. BMC Musculoskelet Disord 2014;15(1):161.

72. Linnstaedt SD, Hu J, Bortsov AV, et al. Mu-opioid receptor gene A118 G variants and persistent pain symptoms among men and women experiencing motor vehicle collision. J Pain 2015;16(7):637–44.

73. Mogil JS, Wilson SG, Chesler EJ, et al. The melanocortin-1 receptor gene mediates female-specific mechanisms of analgesia in mice and humans. Proc Natl Acad Sci U S A 2003;100(8):4867–72.

74. Mannisto PT, Kaakkola S. Catechol-O-methyltransferase (COMT): biochemistry, molecular biology, pharmacology, and clinical efficacy of the new selective COMT inhibitors. Pharmacol Rev 1999;51(4):593–628.

75. Meloto CB, Bortsov AV, Bair E, et al. Modification of COMT-dependent pain sensitivity by psychological stress and sex. Pain 2016;157(4):858–67.

76. Mogil JS, Sorge RE, LaCroix-Fralish ML, et al. Pain sensitivity and vasopressin analgesia are mediated by a gene-sex-environment interaction. Nat Neurosci 2011;14(12):1569–73.

77. Saccò M, Meschi M, Regolisti G, et al. The relationship between blood pressure and pain. J Clin Hypertens 2013;15(8):600–5.

78. Fillingim RB, Maixner W. The influence of resting blood pressure and gender on pain responses. Psychosom Med 1996;58(4):326–32.

79. Myers CD, Robinson ME, Riley JL 3rd, et al. Sex, gender, and blood pressure: contributions to experimental pain report. Psychosom Med 2001;63(4):545–50.

80. Poudevigne MS, O'Connor PJ, Pasley JD. Lack of both sex differences and influence of resting blood pressure on muscle pain intensity. Clin J Pain 2002; 18(6):386–93.

81. Sanford SD, Kersh BC, Thorn BE, et al. Psychosocial mediators of sex differences in pain responsivity. J Pain 2002;3(1):58–64.

82. Thorn BE, Clements KL, Ward LC, et al. Personality factors in the explanation of sex differences in pain catastrophizing and response to experimental pain. Clin J Pain 2004;20(5):275–82.

83. Pool GJ, Schwegler AF, Theodore BR, et al. Role of gender norms and group identification on hypothetical and experimental pain tolerance. Pain 2007; 129(1–2):122–9.

84. Wise EA, Price DD, Myers CD, et al. Gender role expectations of pain: relationship to experimental pain perception. Pain 2002;96(3):335–42.

85. Gijsbers K, Nicholson F. Experimental pain thresholds influenced by sex of experimenter. Percept Mot Skills 2005;101(3):803–7.

86. Kallai I, Barke A, Voss U. The effects of experimenter characteristics on pain reports in women and men. Pain 2004;112(1–2):142–7.

87. Robinson ME, Gagnon CM, Riley JL 3rd, et al. Altering gender role expectations: effects on pain tolerance, pain threshold, and pain ratings. J Pain 2003;4(5): 284–8.
88. Jensen I, Nygren A, Gamberale F, et al. Coping with long-term musculoskeletal pain and its consequences: is gender a factor? Pain 1994;57(2):167–72.
89. Fricchione G. Clinical practice. Generalized anxiety disorder. N Engl J Med 2004;351(7):675–82.
90. Bair MJ, Robinson RL, Katon W, et al. Depression and pain comorbidity: a literature review. Arch Intern Med 2003;163(20):2433–45.
91. Jones A, Zachariae R. Investigation of the interactive effects of gender and psychological factors on pain response. Br J Health Psychol 2004;9(Pt 3): 405–18.
92. Edwards R, Augustson EM, Fillingim R. Sex-specific effects of pain-related anxiety on adjustment to chronic pain. Clin J Pain 2000;16(1):46–53.
93. Stewart SH, Asmundson GJ. Anxiety sensitivity and its impact on pain experiences and conditions: a state of the art. Cogn Behav Ther 2006;35(4):185–8.
94. Hunt C, Keogh E, French CC. Anxiety sensitivity: the role of conscious awareness and selective attentional bias to physical threat. Emotion 2006;6(3): 418–28.
95. Keogh E, Eccleston C. Sex differences in adolescent chronic pain and pain-related coping. Pain 2006;123(3):275–84.
96. Keogh E, Hamid R, Hamid S, et al. Investigating the effect of anxiety sensitivity, gender and negative interpretative bias on the perception of chest pain. Pain 2004;111(1–2):209–17.
97. Keogh E, McCracken LM, Eccleston C. Gender moderates the association between depression and disability in chronic pain patients. Eur J Pain 2006;10(5): 413–22.
98. Unruh AM. Gender variations in clinical pain experience. Pain 1996;65(2–3): 123–67.
99. Shaefer JR, Holland N, Whelan JS, et al. Pain and temporomandibular disorders pharmaco-gender dilemma. Dent Clin North Am 2013;57(2):233–62.
100. LeResche L. Gender disparities in pain. Clin Orthop Relat Res 2011;469(7): 1770–876.
101. Kehlet H, Troels SJ, Clifford JW. Persistent postsurgical pain: risk factors. Lancet 2006;367:1618–25.
102. Greespan JD, Craft RM, LeResche L, et al, the Consensus Working Group on the Sex, Gender, and Pain SIG of the IASP. Studying sex and gender difference in pain and analgesia: a consensus report. Pain 2007;132(Suppl 1):S26–45.
103. Ardakani YH, Rouini MR. Pharmacokinetics of tramadol and its three main metabolites in healthy male and female volunteers. Biopharm Drug Dispos 2007; 28(9):527–34.
104. Backman JT, Schröder MT, Neuvonen PJ. Effects of gender and moderate smoking on the pharmacokinetics and effects of the CYP1A2 substrate tizanidine. Eur J Clin Pharmacol 2008;64(1):17–24.
105. Bendixen KH, Baad-Hansen L, Cairns BE, et al. Effects of low-dose intramuscular ketorolac on experimental pain in the masseter muscle of healthy women. J Orofac Pain 2010;24(4):398–407.
106. Chan S, Edwards SR, Wyse BD, et al. Sex differences in the pharmacokinetics, oxidative metabolism and oral bioavailability of oxycodone in the Sprague-Dawley rat. Clin Exp Pharmacol Physiol 2008;35(3):295–302.

107. Davis AR, Westhoff CL, Stanczyk FZ. Carbamazepine coadministration with an oral contraceptive: effects on steroid pharmacokinetics, ovulation, and bleeding. Epilepsia 2011;52(2):243–7.
108. Ferrari A, Pinetti D, Bertolini A, et al. Interindividual variability of oral sumatriptan pharmacokinetics and of clinical response in migraine patients. Eur J Clin Pharmacol 2008;64(5):489–95.
109. Ferrari A, Tiraferri I, Neri L, et al. Why pharmacokinetic differences among oral triptans have little clinical importance: a comment. J Headache Pain 2011;12(1): 5–12.
110. Granfors MT, Backman JT, Laitila J, et al. Oral contraceptives containing ethinyl estradiol and gestodene markedly increase plasma concentrations and effects of tizanidine by inhibiting cytochrome P450 1A2. Clin Pharmacol Ther 2005; 78(4):400–11.
111. Greenblatt DJ, Harmatz JS, von Moltke LL, et al. Age and gender effects on the pharmacokinetics and pharmacodynamics of triazolam, a cytochrome P450 3A substrate. Clin Pharmacol Ther 2004;76(5):467–79.
112. Lobo ED, Bergstrom RF, Reddy S, et al. In vitro and in vivo evaluations of cytochrome P450 1A2 interactions with duloxetine. Clin Pharmacokinet 2008;47(3): 191–202.
113. McCormack PL, Keating GM. Duloxetine: in stress urinary incontinence. Drugs 2004;64(22):2567–73 [discussion: 2574–5].
114. Nanau RM, Neuman MG. Ibuprofen-induced hypersensitivity syndrome. Transl Res 2010;155(6):275–93.
115. Tsatsaris V, Cabrol D, Carbonne B. Pharmacokinetics of tocolytic agents. Clin Pharmacokinet 2004;43(13):833–44.
116. Wade A, Pawsey S, Whale H, et al. Pharmacokinetics of two 6-day frovatriptan dosing regimens used for the short-term prevention of menstrual migraine: a phase I, randomized, double-blind, placebo-controlled, two-period crossover, single-centre study in healthy female volunteers. Clin Drug Investig 2009; 29(5):325–37.
117. Wegner I, Edelbroek P, de Haan GJ, et al. Drug monitoring of lamotrigine and oxcarbazepine combination during pregnancy. Epilepsia 2010;51(12):2500–2.
118. Wolff K, Boys A, Rostami-Hodjegan A, et al. Changes to methadone clearance during pregnancy. Eur J Clin Pharmacol 2005;61(10):763–8.

Mind-Body Considerations in Orofacial Pain

Hayley A. Cole, MS[a], Charles R. Carlson, PhD, ABPP[b],*

KEYWORDS

- Psychosocial connection • Psychology • Diagnosis • Orofacial pain management

KEY POINTS

- Matched cohort and prospective studies have shown strong associations between OFP and psychological dysfunction. Depression and somatization consistently appear as predictors of OFP onset and maintenance and pain-related disability.
- Sleep quality, parafunctional behaviors, and smoking history serve as important behavioral predictors for TMD development and maintenance.
- Findings suggest there are likely reciprocal relationships between emotions, cognitions, behaviors, and pain experiences for patients with OFP such that dysfunction in one area increases the odds of dysfunction in another.
- Research supports multimodal OFP interventions that address cognitive distortions, self-regulation, and behavioral management.

INTRODUCTION

Orofacial pain (OFP) is a broad term that refers to pain experienced in the face, mouth, or neck. Although a wide variety of disorders can lead to OFP, clinicians and researchers are particularly interested in temporomandibular disorders (TMDs) because they are a frequently experienced and often debilitating class of pain disorders. TMDs are the third most commonly reported chronic pain condition in the world[1] and are estimated to affect between 5%[2] and 10%[3] of the adult population. Some estimates suggest women are up to three times more likely than men to develop a TMD, and TMDs occur more frequently in older adults and non-Hispanic white persons.[4] Despite the high prevalence rates, patients with OFP often find it difficult to receive adequate care. Studies suggest that somewhere between one-half and two-thirds of TMDs fail to remit within 5 years of onset.[4] A recent survey of 101 patients with chronic OFP revealed that on average, patients attended seven consultations with health providers

Disclosure Statement: The authors have nothing to disclose.
[a] Department of Psychology, University of Kentucky, 111 Kastle Hall, Lexington, KY 40506, USA;
[b] Department of Psychology, Orofacial Pain Clinic, University of Kentucky, 209-A Kastle Hall, Lexington, KY 40506, USA
* Corresponding author.
E-mail address: ccarl@email.uky.edu

and saw three specialists to treat their pain; and even then, only 24% of patients classified their treatment as "successful."[5]

OROFACIAL PAIN AND PSYCHOSOCIAL FACTORS

Numerous research groups in the twentieth century demonstrated that OFP is often associated with significant psychological dysfunction. Patients who report OFP symptoms also report higher rates of anxiety and depression than matched non-OFP control subjects.[6–9] Researchers have found strong associations between OFP and trauma. Anonymous patient surveys indicate that 68% of OFP patients report a history of physical or sexual abuse.[10] However, evidence is mixed as to whether or not abuse history relates to pain severity.[10,11] OFP has also been linked to factors associated with general psychological well-being, such as sleep quality,[9] fatigue,[12] self-deception,[12] respiration rate,[7] cardiovascular activity,[13] and emotionality.[13]

Although twentieth century work helped to establish that an association exists between OFP and psychological functioning, most of these studies were limited to correlational work with matched control subjects and thus, researchers were unable to establish temporal relationships between these variables. During this time period, two studies used longitudinal designs to follow patients presenting with TMD and identify psychological factors that differed between patients with acute and chronic TMD.[14,15] Although there was some evidence to suggest depression and somatization relate to TMD chronicity,[15] there was no evidence to suggest that psychological factors predict changes in pain intensity over time.[14]

Together, these studies speak to the idea that OFP likely has physical and psychosocial components. However, the studies stopped short of allowing investigators to determine whether psychological distress is a precursor to OFP, psychological distress is a by-product of dealing with chronic OFP, or co-occurrence is less sequential in nature (eg, both disorders are the consequence of some other variable). As a result, by the end of the twentieth century, the National Institutes of Health consensus conference on TMD management called for the development of conceptual theories and high-quality empirical studies that could clarify the role of psychosocial variables in the development and maintenance of TMDs.[16]

TWENTY-FIRST CENTURY ADVANCEMENTS IN OROFACIAL PAIN: OROFACIAL PAIN: PROSPECTIVE RISK EVALUATION AND ASSESSMENT STUDIES

Heeding the National Institutes of Health TMD conference's call, a group of international scientists initiated The Orofacial Pain: Prospective Risk Evaluation and Assessment (OPPERA) study.[4] The OPPERA study was the first large-scale, prospective study designed to identify biopsychosocial factors that contribute to TMD development and maintenance. The original OPPERA studies spanned 7 years and included a case-control and a prospective cohort study. The case control study matched 185 persons with chronic TMD to 1633 asymptomatic control subjects to identify factors that appeared more frequently in TMD patients than non-TMD patients. The prospective study recruited 2737 volunteers with no past or present TMD diagnoses and followed participants for up to 5 years (mean, 2.8 years) to identify features present at baseline that predicted the development of TMD.[17] Both studies used samples of adults between the ages of 18 and 44 recruited around four large cities in the United States. Taken together, the two studies helped to identify psychological and physiologic factors that seem to contribute to TMD onset and chronicity. Because of the limited scope of this article, only findings most relevant to the relationship between OFP and psychological factors are reported next.

Matched Cohort Study

In accordance with past findings, the OPPERA matched cohort study found there were a variety of psychosocial differences between TMD and TMD-free persons.[18] TMD cases reported higher depression, anxiety, somatization, negative affect, neuroticism, stress, catastrophizing, and hostility scores than TMD-free control subjects. TMD cases reported lower levels of positive affect than control subjects. Somatic awareness (or the tendency to be bothered by common bodily sensations) was the feature that differed most between the two groups, with TMD cases exhibiting standardized odds ratios greater than 2.0, indicating that somatic awareness was significantly associated with the presence of a TMD.

In addition to affective and cognitive variables, the OPPERA study investigated specific behaviors that could be used to differentiate TMD cases from TMD-free control subjects. TMD cases were revealed to have overall poorer quality of sleep than persons with TMD.[18] Parafunctional behaviors (eg, chewing gum) were shown to occur more frequently in patients with TMD than control subjects.[19] Lastly, there were significant differences in smoking behaviors between TMD and TMD-free persons. Although both groups reported similar percentages of current smokers, TMD patients reported more than double the percentage of former smokers as compared with persons who did not report TMD symptoms.

The OPPERA matched cohort study confirmed there are several significant mind and body differences between TMD patients and case control subjects. Although several of these differences had been demonstrated before in prior matched-pairs studies,[7,9] the OPPERA study was able to replicate past results using a large, diverse sample of TMD cases and control subjects recruited from the same community sample to reduce sampling bias. The findings from this study offered support for the hypothesis that heightened somatic awareness, psychological and affective distress, and perceptions of stress may be risk factors for the development of TMD. Similarly, poor sleep, frequent parafunctional behaviors, and a history of smoking may be behaviors that put people at risk for TMD development. However, the cross-sectional nature of the study made it impossible to distinguish whether these factors predisposed healthy people to develop TMD or instead, functioned as symptoms of TMD.[19] Thus, further longitudinal work was needed to help deduce causality.

Prospective Cohort Study

Perhaps the greatest advancements in OFP research to date have come from the OPPERA prospective cohort study. This large-scale, longitudinal study followed initially symptom-free individuals for up to 5 years to allow for identification of psychological and physiologic factors that act as precursors to OFP. Out of the 2737 men and women who provided both baseline and follow-up data, 260 developed OFP during the study. This represents a TMD prevalence rate of approximately 4% in the young to middle age adult population.[20]

The OPPERA prospective cohort study found that several psychological factors can be used to predict first-onset TMD. Consistent with the OPPERA matched-pairs study, TMD cases reported higher scores for all SCL 90R subscales (including depression, anxiety, somatization, obsessive compulsive, hostility, phobia, paranoid, and psychotic), neuroticism, perceived stress, state and trait anxiety, and negative affect. The prospective study also again found that TMD cases reported lower experiences of positive affect. Similar to the matched cohort study, when all significant predictors were entered together in one predictive model, somatic awareness emerged as the strongest predictor of TMD. Although there were many similar findings between the matched-pairs and prospective cohort studies, the prospective study found that symptoms associated with traumatic experiences positively predicted TMD first onset. Furthermore, catastrophizing and coping were not significant predictors of first-onset TMD in the prospective study, despite their long history as predictors of TMD chronicity.

Behavioral differences between TMD and TMD-free persons in the prospective cohort study were similar to those found in the matched-pairs study. In an examination of clinical factors associated with TMD, oral parafunctional behaviors were the strongest predictor of first-onset TMD, with TMD patients reporting more frequent behaviors.[21] This speaks to the role of possible systematic dysregulation in the development of OFP. Poor sleep quality was also shown to be a highly important indicator of TMD onset because it predicted TMD onset even after controlling for a wide range of general health status indicators (including other pain conditions).[22] Lastly, findings again indicated the presence of a relationship between smoking and TMD occurrence; participants who reported a history of smoking at least 100 cigarettes in their lifetime were more likely to develop TMD than participants with no extensive smoking history.

Similar findings across the prospective and matched-pairs studies suggest that the same psychological (particularly somatization) and behavioral factors (including poor sleep and oral parafunctions) contribute to the initial onset and maintenance of TMDs. Thus, when it comes to deducing the temporal relationships between OFP and psychosocial factors, it seems unlikely that experiences of psychological dysfunction and poor sleep are merely consequences of dealing with a chronic pain condition. Instead, it at a minimum suggests that psychological distress has a long-standing, wide-reaching impact on the body and mind that can result in painful TMD experiences many months later.[17] It also lends support to the theory that there are likely reciprocal relationships between emotions, cognitions, behaviors, and pain experiences such that dysfunction in one area increases the odds of dysfunction in another[22]; however, further work is needed to confirm these relationships. In summary, the OPPERA studies suggest that TMD is a complex diagnosis, presumably with multiple causal factors, including but not limited to affective, cognitive, and behavioral dysfunction.[20]

ADDITIONAL LONGITUDINAL STUDIES

Although the OPPERA studies are the most well-known and comprehensive evaluations of OFP to date, additional twenty-first century research groups have conducted longitudinal studies to better understand the development of OFP. Multiple studies have found longitudinal evidence for a relationship between OFP and depression. Liao and colleagues[23] analyzed the health insurance records of nearly 38,000 adults in Taiwan, comparing adults being treated for depression with nondepressed adults. A review of these patients' insurance records over the course of 8 years indicated that depressed patients were 2.7 times more likely than nondepressed patients to develop TMD. In a separate study of general dentistry patients, depression scores at baseline were linked to the development of new-onset chronic OFP 2 years later.[24] The same study found similar relationships between anxiety and somatization and new onset of chronic OFP.

A final study of note explored psychological comorbidities of atypical facial pain.[25] Based on examination, more than half of atypical facial pain patients met diagnostic criteria for a mental disorder. Specifically, 41% of the total sample reported an axis I psychiatric disorder (eg, major depressive disorder, generalized anxiety disorder) that predated their facial pain and 20% of the total sample reported a personality disorder that predated their facial pain. Some caution is warranted in interpreting these results because the study relied on a small sample size (N = 63) and patient self-report for the timeline of symptom onset. However, these findings are in line with the OPPERA prospective study in suggesting that psychological dysfunction, particularly depression and preoccupation with somatic symptoms, likely serve as precursors to the development of chronic and acute OFP for many patients.

PSYCHOLOGICAL DIFFERENTIATORS OF PAIN CHRONICITY AND SEVERITY

Because evidence suggests that less than half of all TMD cases remit within 5 years of onset,[4] identification of factors that can differentiate between chronic and acute TMD cases is important. Recently, investigators have begun to examine whether psychological factors can fulfill this role. Using a sample of Israeli TMD patients, researchers found that chronic TMD patients reported significantly higher levels of depression than acute TMD patients.[26] There were no significant differences between anxiety and somatization for the two groups. In contrast, a large, multisite study of TMD patients did not find evidence to suggest that depression or somatization were related to pain duration.[27] Thus, although there is strong evidence to support that psychological factors relate to OFP onset and maintenance, evidence is mixed as to whether these same factors relate to OFP duration.

Researchers have also investigated psychological variables' ability to predict differences in pain-related disability. Four studies of TMD patients found that depression was predictive of pain-related disability.[24,26,28,29] Although three of the same studies found similar effects for somatization, evidence was mixed as to whether or not anxiety had similar predictive abilities. These findings suggest that patients who experience both TMD and psychological distress (at least in the forms of somatization and depression) may experience pain to be more overwhelming and disabling than patients who experience pain alone.

OROFACIAL PAIN IN CHILDREN AND ADOLESCENTS

As more becomes known about psychological factors related to OFP in adults, researchers have also sought to better understand these processes in children and adolescents. Research has shown that many of the variables predictive of OFP onset and maintenance are similar in adolescents and adults. LeResche and colleagues[30] conducted a 3-year longitudinal study of 1674 11 year olds who reported no TMD pain at baseline. Only 2% of their adolescent sample went on to develop TMD, but those who did reported significantly higher levels of depression and somatization at baseline than TMD-free peers. Contrary to findings in adults,[19,22] adolescents who reported a history of smoking were less likely to report facial pain. Researchers found that the strongest predictor of TMD in adolescents was life satisfaction. Adolescents who reported they were "dissatisfied" with their life at baseline were more than four times more likely than "satisfied" or "highly satisfied" adolescents to develop TMD.

Investigators also explored this sample of adolescents more carefully using latent growth curve analyses.[31] Adolescents were clustered into trajectories by pain intensity and frequency for each of four types of pain complaints (back, head, stomach, and face pain). Adolescents whose trajectories indicated the highest probability of follow-up facial pain had the highest baseline depression and somatization scores of any trajectory group with pain at any site. Furthermore, results again indicated that this group of adolescents prone to facial pain had low life satisfaction.

Exploration of psychological factors predicting TMD in children has been more limited. To date, a small cross-sectional matched cohort study of Brazilian children (ages 8–12) did not find evidence that depressive symptoms differed significantly between children with and without TMD.[32] They did, however, find that anxiety was a strong predictor of TMD; children with high levels of anxiety were 18 times more likely to meet diagnostic criteria for TMD than children with low levels of anxiety.

Together these findings indicate that the relationships between psychological dysfunction and OFP can present early in life. Although the prevalence rates of TMD were low in adolescent populations, many of the mind-body connections present in adulthood were replicated in adolescent samples. Particularly, these findings again solidified the importance of hypervigilance of somatic symptoms in the development of OFP while also introducing the idea that broader psychosocial factors (eg, life satisfaction) may play an important role in early OFP development. At this time, it is unclear whether these early appearing relationships are reflective of genetic influence or early life experiences that have long-lasting impact on future distress and the development of pain.

IMPLICATIONS OF RECENT FINDINGS FOR TREATMENT INTERVENTIONS

Decades of research have revealed that TMD (and more generally, OFP) is a complex, biopsychosocial pain experience. Mounting evidence suggests that many TMDs cannot be conceptualized as a localized OFP condition because they are irreversibly intertwined with psychological, biologic, and behavioral factors. Many of the same factors are associated with both TMD first onset and TMD maintenance, suggesting the probable existence of reciprocal relationships. Factors that may act as precursors to TMD may also act as TMD symptoms once pain begins. Thus, it is useful to consider TMD to be both the result and the cause of multisystem dysfunction. Assessments of and treatments for TMDs must take this same multisystem approach because interventions designed to intervene with only one aspect of the dysfunction (eg, physiologic) are unlikely to be successful. Clinicians and researchers must instead consider a multimodal treatment that corrects dysfunction in patients' thoughts, emotions, behaviors, and physiology.[20]

Multiple investigations have indicated that persons with TMD are characterized by unremitting pain, sleep disturbances, fatigue, and negative emotions (including depression and anxiety).[7,9,17,18,33,34] One way to interpret these findings is that together, these elements represent a failure of self-regulatory control. Pain that persists even long after tissue repair suggests a potential problem in descending inhibitory control systems. Similarly, when sleep onset is delayed or sleep duration is disrupted by frequent awakenings it is likely that a potential source of these disturbances involves a dysregulation of normal inhibitory control systems designed to promote sleep. Perceived fatigue without an identifiable physiologic basis can also be construed as a problem linked to a failure of inhibitory controls. Persistent negative emotions can likewise represent a failure of inhibitory control (cannot stop or switch an ongoing emotional state, which is characteristic of normal adult emotional regulation). Taken together, these findings suggest that persons with TMD may have self-regulatory deficits that manifest in pain, sleep disturbance, fatigue, and psychological distress.[35]

Thayer and Lane[36] have argued that self-regulatory capacity is controlled by the central autonomic network and is indexed by measuring heart rate variability. Offering support for this theory are several investigators' findings that patients with TMD display lower heart rate variability than matched control subjects.[34,37,38] However, in the OPPERA prospective study, heart rate variability did not predict onset of TMD.[39] Only resting heart rate was predictive of TMD onset (those who developed

TMD had higher resting heart rate at the initial evaluation than those that did not). Interventions incorporating strategies that improve heart rate variability have been associated with TMD symptom reductions, which offers further support for the idea that lower heart rate variability in TMD patients may be a factor contributing to the maintenance of the pain.[12]

RECOMMENDATIONS REGARDING OROFACIAL PAIN ASSESSMENT

Before one can intervene with OFP, one must thoroughly assess pain and its many potential contributors and effects. Today the most widely used protocol for research and clinical assessment of TMD is the Diagnostic Criteria for TMD (DC/TMD).[40] This evidence-based assessment protocol uses two axes for comprehensive assessment of TMD. Axis I provides protocols for physical assessment of pain and dysfunction; and axis II provides guidelines for the assessment of psychosocial distress, pain intensity and disability, and parafunctional behaviors. The workgroups involved in the creation of the DC/TMD recognize that, "psychosocial factors are at least as important for the treatment outcome as are initial pain intensity and physical diagnoses"[40(p.17)] and thus suggest that axis II assessment instruments be administered to all TMD patients. More specifically, it is recommended that at a minimum clinicians and researchers screen all patients for pain intensity, pain locations, functioning in response to pain, jaw limitation, distress, and parafunctional behaviors. More comprehensive assessments of patients who endorse evidence of psychosocial dysfunction should be a normal part of initial evaluations so that patients are assessed for depression, anxiety, and additional physical symptoms. It is worth noting that although a comprehensive axis II assessment is time consuming, it has the potential to yield powerful benefits. Past studies of chronic OFP patients have shown that patients' beliefs about pain are one of the most important predictors of treatment outcome.[29] Furthermore, evidence gathered in axis II assessments may allow for important tailoring of patients' treatment. In a recent review of randomized controlled trials of TMD treatment, six of seven studies reviewed found evidence to suggest treatments tailored to patients' unique psychosocial characteristics offered benefits over standardized treatments.[41]

SUPPORT FOR PSYCHOLOGICALLY BASED OROFACIAL PAIN TREATMENTS

Although effective OFP treatment involves psychological and physiologic interventions, strictly physiologic interventions within the dental realm are beyond the scope of this article. Thus, the remainder of this article focuses on briefly reviewing the empirical support for psychologically based treatments of TMD; we review treatments that intervene primarily with patients' affect, cognitions, and specific behaviors. Those interested in medical/dental OFP treatments should see other articles in this issue. Although empirical evidence for psychologically oriented treatments is limited, select interventions have shown substantial promise.

Cognitive behavioral therapy (CBT) treatments have demonstrated efficacy in the treatment of OFP. CBT treatments are based on original psychotherapy models by Beck,[42] which propose that interpretations of events (ie, thoughts) have causal influences on people's emotional experiences and ultimately behaviors; thus, altering one's thoughts can have powerful influence on affects and actions. This theory is particularly important in regards to how OFP patients interpret their pain. Patients who interpret their pain to be debilitating and threatening are likely to experience more psychological distress than those who consider their pain to be aggravating but innocuous. Early work by Dworkin and colleagues[43] revealed that TMD patients who received a brief group-format CBT intervention (focused on education about pain, self-monitoring, relaxation, and coping skills) in addition to their usual treatment reported greater long-term improvements in pain than patients who received only treatment as usual.

Gatchel and colleagues[44] used a more extensive CBT protocol for patients deemed to be at high-risk for progressing from acute to chronic TMDs. Their protocol consisted of six individual CBT sessions (focused on education regarding pain and stress, relaxation training, cognitive restructuring, and implementation of pleasant activities and distraction) in conjunction with biofeedback training. At 1-year follow-up, patients who received the comprehensive CBT/biofeedback treatment reported significantly less pain and symptoms of depression than patients who had not received an intervention. Patients in the "no-intervention" group were considerably more likely to meet criteria for a psychological disorder at follow-up. Additional studies have also found support for the use of CBT treatments for TMD.[45–47]

Although evaluations of CBT suggest that OFP is improved by addressing dysfunctional thoughts, other studies suggest that behavioral interventions can also reduce OFP. Freitas and colleagues[48] conducted a review of seven blind-randomized controlled studies that used counseling and self-management therapies to intervene with OFP. They found that most treatments involved providing patients with an explanation of pain cause; function; contributing psychosocial and physiologic factors; and the benign, or self-limiting nature of the disorder. Self-management therapies varied across studies but most commonly included promotion of rest of facial muscles and joints, reduction of parafunctional habits, and improvement of posture and sleep. The review indicated that splint therapies did not offer any benefits over counseling and self-management therapies; there was some evidence to suggest that physical therapy and postural training in conjunction with self-management therapies may offer select benefits to self-management therapies alone. The authors note that most of the counseling and self-management therapies they reviewed could be conducted by health professionals with little training in psychology, which may make them more accessible to patients and clinicians alike.

One of the protocols reviewed in the meta-analysis involved the physical self-regulation program developed by Carlson and colleagues.[12] This protocol involves the following elements:

- Provide an explanation of the ongoing pain and help patient develop ownership
- Establish rest positions of body structures in trigeminal region
- Monitor head position to avoid tilting and excessive use of motor activity
- Ease upper back tightness
- Take brief relaxation breaks using empirically validated behavioral relaxation protocol
- Begin sleep in relaxed position using the postural positions introduced in relaxation protocol
- Exercise and drink fluids regularly; develop regular program of activity improving aerobic capacity and ensuring adequate hydration
- Entrain diaphragmatic breathing pattern to a criterion of three to seven breaths per minute when actively attempting to relax

These activities are introduced to patients over three 50-minute sessions and have been demonstrated to reduce pain symptoms by almost 70% at 6-month follow-up. The physical self-regulation approach incorporates elements from the work of others and demonstrates how a multimodal treatment intervention exerts important and durable outcomes.

Heart rate variability has a potential role as a measure of self-regulatory capacity. It is therefore not surprising that effective self-management therapies include relaxation training and diaphragmatic breathing training.[12] Both of these skill sets involve enhancing parasympathetic control with behaviorally based interventions directly influencing measures of heart rate variability and in particular, measures of high-frequency heart rate variability. Note that for these interventions to have the desired influence on parasympathetic tone the individual needs to master the performance of the skill sets. In the case of relaxation training, for example, individuals must be able to maintain a set of relaxed positions and focused attention to promote parasympathetic tone. Similarly, diaphragmatic breathing training to criteria (eg, minimal chest movement; respiration rate of three to seven breaths per minute; and self-reports of a positive, relaxed state) is needed to obtain the maximum benefit for enhancing parasympathetic activity. This suggests that an important component of behaviorally based skills training is to ensure participants engage in the learning and practice of the skills to criterion-based levels of competency.

SUMMARY

This article reviews and summarizes the cognitive, behavioral, and emotional factors that contribute to the onset and maintenance of chronic TMDs, and discusses the cognitive and behavioral treatment of TMDs. These OFP conditions illustrate the dynamic interplay of the mind and body and the importance of multimodal treatment approaches addressing simultaneously the cognitive, behavioral, and physiologic dimensions of facial pain. One of the challenges of modern health care is to provide patients with timely access to providers from different perspectives with different skill sets to address complex conditions having multiple mind-body interactions. Effective management of TMD can best be obtained by interprofessional care guided by a biopsychosocial perspective that addresses fully the relationships between the mind and the body.

REFERENCES

1. Dworkin SF. Temporomandibular disorder (TMD) pain–related disability found related to depression, nonspecific physical symptoms, and pain duration at 3 international sites. J Evid Based Dent Pract 2011;11(3):143–4.
2. Isong U, Gansky SA, Plesh O. Temporomandibular joint and muscle disorder-type pain in US adults: the National Health Interview Survey. J Orofac Pain 2008;22(4): 317–22.
3. Janal M, Raphael K, Nayak S, et al. Prevalence of myofascial temporomandibular disorder in US community women. J Oral Rehabil 2008;35(11):801–9.
4. Maixner W, Diatchenko L, Dubner R, et al. Orofacial pain prospective evaluation and risk assessment study: the OPPERA study. J Pain 2011;12(11 Suppl):T4.
5. Beecroft E, Durham J, Thomson P. Retrospective examination of the healthcare 'journey' of chronic orofacial pain patients referred to oral and maxillofacial surgery. Br Dent J 2013;214(5):E12.
6. McCreary CP, Clark GT, Merril RL, et al. Psychological distress and diagnostic subgroups of temporomandibular disorder patients. Pain 1991;44(1): 29–34.
7. Curran SL, Carlson CR, Okeson JP. Emotional and physiologic responses to laboratory challenges: patients with temporomandibular disorders versus matched control subjects. J Orofac Pain 1996;10(2):141–50.

8. Korszun A, Hinderstein B, Wong M, et al. Comorbidity of depression with chronic facial pain and temporomandibular disorders. Oral Surg Oral Med Oral Pathol Oral Radiol Endod 1996;82(5):496–500.

9. Carlson CR, Reid KI, Curran SL, et al. Psychological and physiological parameters of masticatory muscle pain. Pain 1998;76(3):297–307.

10. Curran SL, Sherman JJ, Cunningham LL, et al. Physical and sexual abuse among orofacial pain patients: linkages with pain and psychologic distress. J Orofacial Pain 1995;9(4):340–6.

11. Fillingim RB, Maixner W, Sigurdsson A, et al. Sexual and physical abuse history in subjects with temporomandibular disorders: relationship to Cl cal variables, pain sensitivity, and psychologic factors. J Orofac Pain 1997;11(1):48–57.

12. Carlson CR, Bertrand PM, Ehrlich AD, et al. Physical self-regulation training for the management of temporomandibular disorders. J Orofac Pain 2001;15(1): 47–55.

13. Carlson CR, Okeson JP, Falace DA, et al. Comparison of psychologic and physiologic functioning between patients with masticatory muscle pain and matched controls. J Orofac Pain 1993;7(1):15–22.

14. Ohrbach R, Dworkin SF. Five-year outcomes in TMD: relationship of changes in pain to changes in physical and psychological variables. Pain 1998;74(2): 315–26.

15. Garofalo JP, Gatchel RJ, Wesley AL, et al. Predicting chronicity in acute temporomandibular joint disorders using the research diagnostic criteria. J Am Dent Assoc 1998;129(4):438–47.

16. Albino J, Beck J, Berkley K, et al. Management of temporomandibular disorders. J Am Dental Assoc 1996;127(11):1595–606.

17. Fillingim RB, Ohrbach R, Greenspan JD, et al. Psychological factors associated with development of TMD: the OPPERA prospective cohort study. J Pain 2013; 14(12):T75–90.

18. Fillingim RB, Ohrbach R, Greenspan JD, et al. Potential psychosocial risk factors for chronic TMD: descriptive data and empirically identified domains from the OPPERA case-control study. J Pain 2011;12(11):T46–60.

19. Ohrbach R, Fillingim RB, Mulkey F, et al. Clinical findings and pain symptoms as potential risk factors for chronic TMD: descriptive data and empirically identified domains from the OPPERA case-control study. J Pain 2011;12(11):T27–45.

20. Slade GD, Fillingim RB, Sanders AE, et al. Summary of findings from the OPPERA prospective cohort study of incidence of first-onset temporomandibular disorder: implications and future directions. J Pain 2013;14(12):T116–24.

21. Ohrbach R, Bair E, Fillingim RB, et al. Clinical orofacial characteristics associated with risk of first-onset TMD: the OPPERA prospective cohort study. J Pain 2013; 14(12):T33–50.

22. Sanders AE, Slade GD, Bair E, et al. General health status and incidence of first-onset temporomandibular disorder: the OPPERA prospective cohort study. J Pain 2013;14(12):T51–62.

23. Liao CH, Chang CS, Chang SN, et al. The risk of temporomandibular disorder in patients with depression: a population-based cohort study. Community Dent Oral Epidemiol 2011;39(6):525–31.

24. Aggarwal VR, Macfarlane GJ, Farragher TM, et al. Risk factors for onset of chronic oro-facial pain: results of the North Cheshire oro-facial pain prospective population study. Pain 2010;149(2):354–9.

25. Taiminen T, Kuusalo L, Lehtinen L, et al. Psychiatric (axis I) and personality (axis II) disorders in patients with burning mouth syndrome or atypical facial pain. Scand J Pain 2011;2(4):155–60.

26. Reiter S, Emodi-Perlman A, Goldsmith C, et al. Comorbidity between depression and anxiety in patients with temporomandibular disorders according to the research diagnostic criteria for temporomandibular disorders. J Oral Facial Pain Headache 2015;29(2):135–43.

27. Manfredini D, Winocur E, Ahlberg J, et al. Psychosocial impairment in temporomandibular disorders patients. RDC/TMD axis II findings from a multicentre study. J Dent 2010;38(10):765–72.

28. Ozdemir-Karatas M, Peker K, Balık A, et al. Identifying potential predictors of pain–related disability in Turkish patients with chronic temporomandibular disorder pain. J Headache Pain 2013;14(1):17.

29. Galli U, Ettlin DA, Palla S, et al. Do illness perceptions predict pain-related disability and mood in chronic orofacial pain patients? A 6-month follow-up study. Eur J Pain 2010;14(5):550–8.

30. LeResche L, Mancl LA, Drangsholt MT, et al. Predictors of onset of facial pain and temporomandibular disorders in early adolescence. Pain 2007;129(3):269–78.

31. Dunn KM, Jordan KP, Mancl L, et al. Trajectories of pain in adolescents: a prospective cohort study. Pain 2011;152(1):66–73.

32. Pizolato RA, Freitas-Fernandes FSD, Gavião MBD. Anxiety/depression and orofacial myofacial disorders as factors associated with TMD in children. Braz Oral Res 2013;27(2):156–62.

33. Carlson CR, Okeson JP, Falace DA, et al. Stretch-based relaxation and the reduction of EMG activity among masticatory muscle pain patients. J Craniomandib Disord 1991;5(3):205–12.

34. Schmidt JE, Carlson CR. A controlled comparison of emotional reactivity and physiological response in masticatory muscle pain patients. J Orofac Pain 2009;23(3):230–42.

35. Sauer SE, Burris JL, Carlson CR. New directions in the management of chronic pain: self-regulation theory as a model for integrative clinical psychology practice. Clin Psychol Rev 2010;30(6):805–14.

36. Thayer JF, Lane RD. A model of neurovisceral integration in emotion regulation and dysregulation. J Affect Disord 2000;61(3):201–16.

37. Nes LS, Carlson CR, Crofford LJ, et al. Self-regulatory deficits in fibromyalgia and temporomandibular disorders. Pain 2010;151(1):37–44.

38. Maixner W, Greenspan JD, Dubner R, et al. Potential autonomic risk factors for chronic TMD: descriptive data and empirically identified domains from the OPPERA case-control study. J Pain 2011;12(11):T75–91.

39. Greenspan JD, Slade GD, Bair E, et al. Pain sensitivity and autonomic factors associated with development of TMD: the OPPERA prospective cohort study. J Pain 2013;14(12):T63–74, e66.

40. Schiffman E, Ohrbach R, Truelove E, et al. Diagnostic criteria for temporomandibular disorders (DC/TMD) for clinical and research applications: recommendations of the International RDC/TMD Consortium Network and Orofacial Pain Special Interest Group. J Oral Facial Pain Headache 2014;28(1):6–27.

41. Kotiranta U, Suvinen T, Forssell H. Tailored treatments in temporomandibular disorders: where are we now? A systematic qualitative literature review. J Oral Facial Pain Headache 2014;28(1):28–37.

42. Beck JS. Cognitive behavior therapy: basics and beyond. New York: Guilford Press; 2011.

43. Dworkin SF, Turner JA, Wilson L, et al. Brief group cognitive-behavioral intervention for temporomandibular disorders. Pain 1994;59(2):175–87.

44. Gatchel RJ, Stowell AW, Wildenstein L, et al. Efficacy of an early intervention for patients with acute temporomandibular disorder–related pain: a one-year outcome study. J Am Dental Assoc 2006;137(3):339–47.

45. Turk DC, Rudy TE, Kubinski JA, et al. Dysfunctional patients with temporomandibular disorders: evaluating the efficacy of a tailored treatment protocol. J Consult Clin Psychol 1996;64(1):139–46.

46. Turner JA, Mancl L, Aaron LA. Short-and long-term efficacy of brief cognitive-behavioral therapy for patients with chronic temporomandibular disorder pain: a randomized, controlled trial. Pain 2006;121(3):181–94.

47. Litt MD, Shafer DM, Kreutzer DL. Brief cognitive-behavioral treatment for TMD pain: long-term outcomes and moderators of treatment. Pain 2010;151(1):110–6.

48. Freitas R, Ferreira M, Barbosa G, et al. Counselling and self-management therapies for temporomandibular disorders: a systematic review. J Oral Rehabil 2013; 40(11):864–74.

UNITED STATES POSTAL SERVICE®

Statement of Ownership, Management, and Circulation
(All Periodicals Publications Except Requester Publications)

1 Publication Title	2 Publication Number	3 Filing Date
DENTAL CLINICS OF NORTH AMERICA	566 – 480	9/18/2018

4 Issue Frequency	5 Number of Issues Published Annually	6 Annual Subscription Price
JAN, APR, JUL, OCT	4	$294.00

7 Complete Mailing Address of Known Office of Publication (Not printer) (Street, city, county, state, and ZIP+4®)

ELSEVIER INC.
230 Park Avenue, Suite 800
New York, NY 10169

Contact Person
STEPHEN R. BUSHING

Telephone (Include area code)
215-239-3688

8 Complete Mailing Address of Headquarters or General Business Office of Publisher (Not printer)

ELSEVIER INC.
230 Park Avenue, Suite 800
New York, NY 10169

9 Full Names and Complete Mailing Addresses of Publisher, Editor, and Managing Editor (Do not leave blank)

Publisher (Name and complete mailing address)

TAYLOR E. BALL, ELSEVIER INC.
1600 JOHN F KENNEDY BLVD. SUITE 1800
PHILADELPHIA, PA 19103-2899

Editor (Name and complete mailing address)

JOHN VASSALLO, ELSEVIER INC.
1600 JOHN F KENNEDY BLVD. SUITE 1800
PHILADELPHIA, PA 19103-2899

Managing Editor (Name and complete mailing address)

PATRICK MANLEY, ELSEVIER INC.
1600 JOHN F KENNEDY BLVD. SUITE 1800
PHILADELPHIA, PA 19103-2899

10 Owner (Do not leave blank. If the publication is owned by a corporation, give the name and address of the corporation immediately followed by the names and addresses of all stockholders owning or holding 1 percent or more of the total amount of stock. If not owned by a corporation, give the names and addresses of the individual owners. If owned by a partnership or other unincorporated firm, give its name and address as well as those of each individual owner. If the publication is published by a nonprofit organization, give its name and address.)

Full Name	Complete Mailing Address
WHOLLY OWNED SUBSIDIARY OF REED/ELSEVIER, US HOLDINGS	1600 JOHN F KENNEDY BLVD. SUITE 1800 PHILADELPHIA, PA 19103-2899

11 Known Bondholders, Mortgagees, and Other Security Holders Owning or Holding 1 Percent or More of Total Amount of Bonds, Mortgages, or Other Securities. If none, check box. ► ☐ None

Full Name	Complete Mailing Address
N/A	

12 Tax Status (For completion by nonprofit organizations authorized to mail at nonprofit rates) (Check one)
The purpose, function, and nonprofit status of this organization and the exempt status for federal income tax purposes:
☒ Has Not Changed During Preceding 12 Months
☐ Has Changed During Preceding 12 Months (Publisher must submit explanation of change with this statement)

PS Form **3526**, July 2014 [Page 1 of 4 (see instructions page 4)] PSN: 7530-01-000-9931   PRIVACY NOTICE: See our privacy policy on www.usps.com.

---

13 Publication Title	14 Issue Date for Circulation Data Below
DENTAL CLINICS OF NORTH AMERICA	JULY 2018

15 Extent and Nature of Circulation		Average No. Copies Each Issue During Preceding 12 Months	No. Copies of Single Issue Published Nearest to Filing Date
a. Total Number of Copies (Net press run)		291	392
b. Paid Circulation (By Mail and Outside the Mail)	(1) Mailed Outside-County Paid Subscriptions Stated on PS Form 3541 (Include paid distribution above nominal rate, advertiser's proof copies, and exchange copies)	137	169
	(2) Mailed In-County Paid Subscriptions Stated on PS Form 3541 (Include paid distribution above nominal rate, advertiser's proof copies, and exchange copies)	0	0
	(3) Paid Distribution Outside the Mails Including Sales Through Dealers and Carriers, Street Vendors, Counter Sales, and Other Paid Distribution Outside USPS®	103	149
	(4) Paid Distribution by Other Classes of Mail Through the USPS (e.g., First-Class Mail®)	0	0
c. Total Paid Distribution (Sum of 15b (1), (2), (3), and (4))		240	318
d. Free or Nominal Rate Distribution (By Mail and Outside the Mail)	(1) Free or Nominal Rate Outside-County Copies included on PS Form 3541	41	62
	(2) Free or Nominal Rate In-County Copies Included on PS Form 3541	0	0
	(3) Free or Nominal Rate Copies Mailed at Other Classes Through the USPS (e.g., First-Class Mail)	0	0
	(4) Free or Nominal Rate Distribution Outside the Mail (Carriers or other means)	0	0
e. Total Free or Nominal Rate Distribution (Sum of 15d (1), (2), (3) and (4))		41	62
f. Total Distribution (Sum of 15c and 15e)		281	380
g. Copies not Distributed (See Instructions to Publishers #4 (page #3))		10	12
h. Total (Sum of 15f and g)		291	392
i. Percent Paid (15c divided by 15f times 100)		85.41%	83.68%

* If you are claiming electronic copies, go to line 16 on page 3. If you are not claiming electronic copies, skip to line 17 on page 3.

16 Electronic Copy Circulation		Average No. Copies Each Issue During Preceding 12 Months	No. Copies of Single Issue Published Nearest to Filing Date
a. Paid Electronic Copies	►	0	0
b. Total Paid Print Copies (Line 15c) + Paid Electronic Copies (Line 16a)	►	240	318
c. Total Print Distribution (Line 15f) + Paid Electronic Copies (Line 16a)	►	281	380
d. Percent Paid (Both Print & Electronic Copies) (16b divided by 16c × 100)	►	85.41%	83.68%

☒ I certify that 50% of all my distributed copies (electronic and print) are paid above a nominal price.

17 Publication of Statement of Ownership

☒ If the publication is a general publication, publication of this statement is required. Will be printed in the OCTOBER 2018 issue of this publication.   ☐ Publication not required.

18 Signature and Title of Editor, Publisher, Business Manager or Owner

STEPHEN R. BUSHING – INVENTORY DISTRIBUTION CONTROL MANAGER

Stephen R. Bushing   Date 9/18/2018

I certify that all information furnished on this form is true and complete. I understand that anyone who furnishes false or misleading information on this form or who omits material or information requested on the form may be subject to criminal sanctions (including fines and imprisonment) and/or civil sanctions (including civil penalties).

PS Form **3526**, July 2014 (Page 3 of 4)   PRIVACY NOTICE: See our privacy policy on www.usps.com.

Moving?

Make sure your subscription moves with you!

To notify us of your new address, find your **Clinics Account Number** (located on your mailing label above your name), and contact customer service at:

Email: journalscustomerservice-usa@elsevier.com

800-654-2452 (subscribers in the U.S. & Canada)
314-447-8871 (subscribers outside of the U.S. & Canada)

Fax number: 314-447-8029

Elsevier Health Sciences Division
Subscription Customer Service
3251 Riverport Lane
Maryland Heights, MO 63043

*To ensure uninterrupted delivery of your subscription, please notify us at least 4 weeks in advance of move.

ELSEVIER

Printed and bound by CPI Group (UK) Ltd, Croydon, CR0 4YY

03/10/2024

01040849-0007